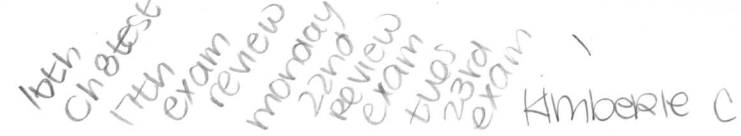
Workbook

Laboratory Testing *for* Ambulatory Settings: A Guide for Health Care Professionals

Second Edition

Marti Garrels, MSA, MT (ASCP), CMA (AAMA)
Medical Assisting Program Director
Lake Washington Technical College
Kirkland, Washington

Carol S. Oatis, MSEd, MT SM (ASCP), CMA (AAMA)
Microbiology Adjunct Instructor
Lake Sumter Community College
Leesburg, Florida

D1402613

ELSEVIER
SAUNDERS

ELSEVIER
SAUNDERS

3251 Riverport Lane
St. Louis, Missouri 63043

WORKBOOK FOR LABORATORY TESTING FOR AMBULATORY SETTINGS: ISBN: 978-1-4377-1908-6
A GUIDE FOR HEALTH CARE PROFESSIONALS

ISBN-13: 978-1-4377-1908-6

Executive Editor: Susan Cole
Developmental Editor: Jennifer Bertucci
Publishing Services Manager: Catherine Jackson
Senior Project Manager: David Stein
Project Manager: Priya Dauntess
Design Direction: Teresa McBryan

Printed in the United States of America

Last digit is the print number: 9   8   7   6   5   4   3   2   1

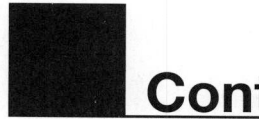# Contents

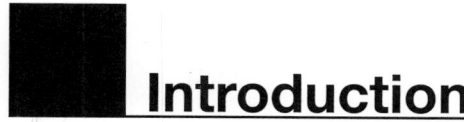# Introduction

This workbook is designed to build mastery over the highly technical and fascinating field of laboratory medicine. Most chapters are organized into five sections: terminology exercises; review questions for fundamental concepts, procedures, advanced concepts; and check-off procedure sheets for all the procedures presented in the textbook chapter. The completed workbook exercises and check-off procedure sheets fulfill all the competency objectives listed at the beginning of each chapter in the textbook. The appendix of the workbook contains laboratory maintenance logs, report forms, quality control logs, patient logs, and a sample health screening assessment form. These forms provide the documentation needed to prove laboratory quality assurance, safety compliance, and proper charting of test results.

TIPS FOR MASTERING EACH CHAPTER

Terminology Exercises

Before reading each chapter, you should become familiar with the technical terms related to the subject. The Evolve Web site provides tutorial exercises using these terms, and the matching exercises in this workbook can help you learn the terms. Making flashcards of the terms is also recommended. As you read the text and fill in your structured notes (from the Evolve Web site), you will find each of the terms bolded and defined in context to reinforce and build further understanding.

Basic Concepts, Procedures, and Advanced Concepts: Review Questions and Labeling

The questions, pictures, and diagrams in these three sections fulfill the stated objectives for each chapter. The questions are designed to follow the textbook and structured notes from the Evolve Web site. You are encouraged to use the textbook alongside the workbook for visual reinforcement and as a reference for finding data from the tables and flow charts. The advanced concepts sections contain complex critical-thinking exercises, as well as referencing detailed laboratory test information in chapters 3 through 9. Your course instructor may assign one or more of these three sections, depending on the time frame of the course.

Check-off Procedure Sheets

The outcome-based procedure sheets are found at the end of each chapter. You are encouraged to locate in the textbook the corresponding procedure box, which provides pictures of the steps involved in each procedure. The procedures fall into two categories: *Skill Procedures,* such as using a microscope, instructing patients, collecting specimens, and staining slides, and *Analytical Tests* in which you follow a test procedure to obtain test results, such as urinalysis, hemoglobin, glucose, and strep tests. In both cases, it is essential that you read, perform, and check off each step on the sheet as satisfactory or unsatisfactory. The steps marked with an asterisk (*) are critical for demonstrating competency. The *Skill Procedures* usually are performed with the instructor verifying each step. The *Analytical Tests* may be performed with a laboratory partner verifying the steps leading up to the test result. The instructor then verifies the final test result and the proper documentation of the test result to fulfill the required measurable outcome.

1 Introduction to the Laboratory and Safety Training

VOCABULARY REVIEW

Match each definition with the correct term.

_c_ 1. Most of the population will test within a range of similar results when testing an analyte

_k_ 2. Laboratory orders indicating what tests are to be done

_b_ 3. A steady state of internal chemical and physical balance

_h_ 4. The substance being tested, such as glucose or cholesterol, in a body specimen

_i_ 5. A test result indicating a threat to a patient's health

_e_ 6. The patient's willingness to follow the treatment plan and take an active role in his or her own health care

_f_ 7. Tests that provide simple, unvarying results and require a minimal amount of judgment and interpretation

_l_ 8. Clotting ability of blood

_m_ 9. A facility or an area within a medical setting in which materials or specimens from the human body are examined or analyzed

_a_ 10. The inability to regulate blood sugar levels

_g_ 11. Long-lasting, debilitating conditions

_d_ 12. Disease-causing microorganisms

_j_ 13. Outpatient health care setting in which patients are not bedridden

A. diabetes mellitus
B. homeostasis
C. reference range
D. pathogens
E. compliance
F. CLIA waived tests
G. chronic disorders
H. analyte
I. critical value
J. ambulatory care
K. requisitions
L. coagulation
M. clinical laboratory

Identify the following acronyms.

14. POCT _Point of care Testing (bedside testing)_

15. CBC _Complete blood count_

16. POL _Physicians office Laboratory_

FUNDAMENTAL CONCEPTS

Overview of the Laboratory

17. List the three reasons a physician would prescribe a laboratory test.

- to screen patients for possible disorders.   screen
- to establish a diagnosis.   comfirm
- to monitor the patient's condition or treatment.   monitor

18. List the three ways a specimen is analyzed.

measuring levels of analytes and comparing to reference values.

Observing and detecting abnormal cells under a microscope.

Detecting the presence of pathogenic microorganisms.

19. List the three types of medical laboratories.

Reference/referral laboratories

Hospital laboratory

Ambulatory Care Setting

20. List three examples of professional credentials (or titles) obtained by individuals who perform laboratory tests based on their educational background (see Table 1-1 in the textbook).

Doctorate: 8 or more years of education	Master: 6 or more years of education	Bachelor: 4 or more years of education	Associate: 1 to 2 years of education
board-certified pathologists	MD	CLS	MLT
MD	DO	MT	CMA
DO	ND	RMT	RMA

21. List three important characteristics required of laboratory personnel.

Professional attitude

motivation

manual dexterity.

22. Give three reasons why a physician would want a test performed in the office and three reasons the specimen would be tested at an outside laboratory.

Advantages of In-Office Testing	Advantages of Out-of-Office Testing
patients can now get results right away.	80% of final diagnoses comes from the lab test.
physicians interpretation and therapeutic can be given on same visit.	patient testing in the hospitals called POCT (bedside and its immediate results)
Basic microscopic procedures that have been CLIA approved.	PCA transmits the results to data management system.
—improves patient compliance	— results can go directly to medical record.

23. From the reference laboratory requisition form (see Figure 1-6 in the textbook), write the first three laboratory tests listed in the following categories for blood, and provide the procedure code and blood collection container.

Test Category	Reference Laboratory Tests (see Requisition)	CPT Code (Left of Test)	Container (Right of Test)
Hematology tests	CBC W DIFF	85025	LAV
	CBC W/O DIFF	85027	LAV
	Hematocrit	85014	LAV
Chemistry tests	Albumin	82040	SST
	Alkaline Phosphatase	84075	SST
	ALT (SGPT)	84460	SST
Serology/immunology tests	ABO and Rh	85610 / 85730	LAV
	Antinuclear antibodies	86038	SST
	Helicobacter pylori, IgG	86677	SST

24. Give the metric unit and abbreviation for each basic unit of measurement.

Measurement	Metric Unit	Abbreviation
Weight	gram	g OR gm
Length	meter	m
Volume (capacity)	liter	l OR L OR cc

25. Give the metric prefix and abbreviation for each of the following.

Fractions	Prefix	Abbreviation
1/10, or 0.1	deci-	d
1/100, or 0.01	centi-	c
1/1000, or 0.001	milli-	m
1/1,000,000, or 0.000001	micro-	mc

26. The following laboratory supplies have temperature storage directions on them. Where should they be stored?

Store at 15° to 30° C ___ROOM___

Store at 0° C ___FREEZER___

Store at 4° to 8° C ___Refrigerator___

prophylaxis

27. Give the military times for the following Greenwich times.

3:00 PM _____15 00_____

8:35 AM _____08 35_____

9:15 PM _____21 15_____

Noon _____12 00_____

Safety

___d___ 28. A documented plan provided by a facility to eliminate or minimize occupational exposure to bloodborne pathogens

___a___ 29. Danger related to the exposure to toxic, unstable, explosive, or flammable materials

___i___ 30. A means of transporting an infectious agent or pathogen from the infected individual to another by air, food, hand-to-hand contact, insects, or body fluids

___g___ 31. The assumption that the blood or body fluid containing blood from any patient or test kit could be infectious

___c___ 32. A disease that is spread within a health care facility

___m___ 33. Federal law protecting employees' right to know about the dangers of the hazardous chemicals they may be exposed to under normal working conditions

___e___ 34. Through the skin

___n___ 35. An area that has been in contact with materials or environmental surfaces where infectious organisms may reside

___l___ 36. Specialized clothing or equipment worn by an employee for protection against infectious materials

___k___ 37. Efforts and research toward isolating and removing bloodborne pathogens from the workplace

___o___ 38. Danger related to exposure to infectious and bloodborne pathogens

___j___ 39. Dangers related to electricity, fire, weather emergencies, bomb threats, and accidental injuries

___f___ 40. Policies that are recorded, monitored, and evaluated to protect employees from exposure to the pathogens in blood or body fluids

___h___ 41. Putting on clothing or equipment as a barrier to a hazard

___b___ 42. CDC recommendations for infection control in health facilities

A. chemical hazard
B. standard precautions
C. nosocomial infection (HCAI)
D. exposure control plan
E. percutaneous
F. work practice controls
G. universal precautions
H. donning personal protective equipment
I. transmission
J. physical hazards
K. engineering controls
L. personal protective equipment
M. hazard communication standard
N. contaminated
O. biohazards

43. List three ways that pathogens (infectious organisms) are transmitted.

_____-by air_____

_____-by insects_____

_____-by bodily fluids_____

44. List three methods to sanitize hands. (Hint: Each uses a different cleanser.)

   washing your hands with Regular soap.

   washing your hands with antimicrobial soap.

   hand Rubbing with alcohol-based hand rub. (most effective)

45. Label the following personal protective equipment.

a goggles

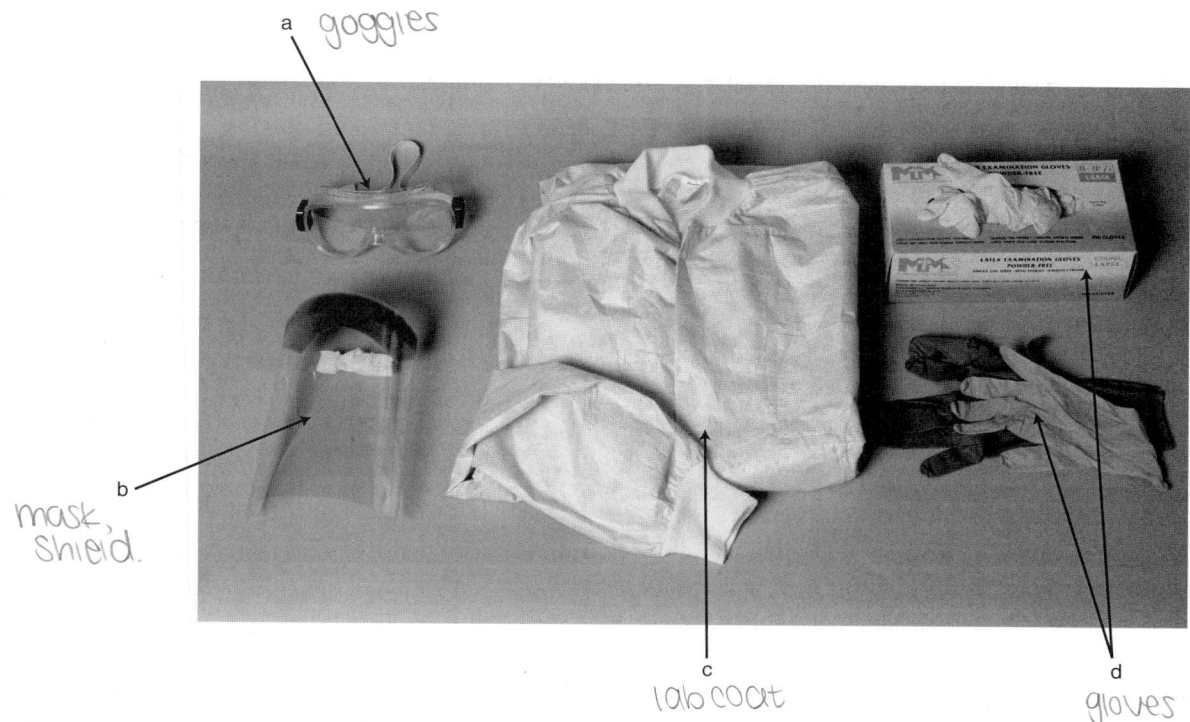

b

mask, shield.

c

lab coat

d

gloves

46. In which of the following disposal containers would contaminated gloves be disposed: wastebasket, biohazard waste container, or biohazard sharps container?

   It will be in the biohazard waste container.

47. List the three major bloodborne pathogens. (Hint: They are all viral.)

   HIV

   Hepatitis B (most prevalent / vaccine)

   Hepatitis C (likely to reach chronic stage later in life)

Hep A (enters through gastrointestinal tracts + attacks liver)

48. Identify the following acronyms related to the bloodborne pathogen standard.

   HCAIs   Health care associated infections

   OPIM   Other potentially infectious materials.

   PPE   Personal protective equipment.

   PEP   Postexposure prophylaxis

49. Identify the following acronyms related to chemical hazard training.

MSDS __material Safety Data Sheet__

NFPA __National Fire Protective Association__

HMIS __Hazardous materials Information System.__

50. List three safety rules that must be observed in the laboratory, and explain why.

- Do not eat, drink, smoke, or apply makeup in areas of exposure.
- Sanitize the hands on and after removing gloves.
- Label all biohazard containers and appliances

51. Use the Internet to locate and identify any OSHA or CDC updates on laboratory safety.

25 States and 2 U.S Territories have their own OSHA-approved occupational safety and health standards.

Procedure 1-1: Proper Use of Personal Protective Equipment

Person evaluated _Kimberle Cornelius_ Date _____

Evaluated by _____ Score _____

Outcome goal	Demonstrate the proper use of personal protective equipment

Conditions	Given the following supplies:
	  hand sanitizer
	  nonpowdered gloves
	  fluid-impenetrable gowns with cuffs at the wrists
	  face masks and goggles, or full face shield (if the procedure to be performed has the
	    potential for splashing)

Standards	Required time: 10 minutes Performance time _____ Total possible points = _____ Points earned = _____

Evaluation Rubric Codes:
S = Satisfactory, meets standard **U** = Unsatisfactory, fails to meet standard

Preparation	Scores	
	S	U
1. Before **donning** (putting on) PPE, remember to perform the hand wash or hand rub appropriately.		

Procedure	Scores	
	S	U
2. Follow the proper sequence for donning PPE.		
a. Put on the gown.		
b. Put on any face protectors.		
c. Don disposable nonsterile, nonpowdered, nonlatex, well-fitting gloves.		
d. Extend the gloves over the gown cuffs.		
3. Keep gloved hands away from the face. Remove gloves if they become torn, and perform hand hygiene before donning new gloves. Avoid touching other surfaces and items not involved in the testing process. The outside of the front of the gown is considered contaminated. The "clean" areas of the gown and gloves are on the inside and the back of the gown.		
4. Sequence for removing PPE:		
a. Properly take off gloves as follows:		
Remove one glove by grasping the outside with the other gloved hand and pulling it off.		
Wad up the removed glove in the gloved hand. Slip an ungloved finger under the cuff and fold it over until you can grasp the inside area of the second glove.		
Pull off the second glove inside-out with the first glove still inside.		
b. Remove the face shield.		
c. Remove the gown.		

Chapter **1** **Introduction to the Laboratory and Safety Training**

Follow-up	Scores	
	S	U
5. If the gloves have visible blood or body fluid on them, dispose of them in a biohazard waste receptacle.		
6. Perform hand hygiene (hand wash or hand rub) immediately after removing PPE.		
Total Points per Column		

2 Regulations, Microscope Setup, and Quality Assurance

VOCABULARY REVIEW

Match each definition with the correct term.

_f_ 1. Tests that produce a result measured as a number

_g_ 2. A substance or ingredient used in a laboratory test to detect, measure, examine, or produce a reaction

_b_ 3. An *overall* process to aid in improving the reliability, efficiency, and quality of laboratory test results

_i_ 4. Materials with known values of the substance measured that help the laboratory achieve accurate and reliable testing by checking if the test system is working

_a_ 5. Instructions included by the manufacturer located in the kit or test package

_h_ 6. Proving competency by testing a specimen from an outside accreditation agency

_c_ 7. Tests that simply look for the presence or absence of a substance

_d_ 8. A process in which known samples (controls) are routinely tested to establish the reliability, accuracy, and precision of a specific test system

_e_ 9. All components of a test that are packaged together

_q_ 10. A built-in positive control to prove the device or test kit is working

_l_ 11. The awareness and prevention of both the physical and procedural risks that may bring about an injury or legal action against the practice

_m_ 12. A pattern of narrow and wide bars and spaces; each pattern is encoded with its own particular meaning

_n_ 13. When both accuracy and precision are accomplished

_R_ 14. Liquid positive and negative controls that are tested the same way as the liquid patient specimen

_p_ 15. Ability to produce the same test result each time a test is performed (results are seen clustered together on a target)

_s_ 16. The average test result of a series of controls

_o_ 17. A statistical term describing the amount of variation from the mean in a dataset

_j_ 18. When controls consistently fall within the two standard deviations of the mean (results are seen within the center of a target)

_k_ 19. Used to plot the daily results of the control samples

A. package insert
B. quality assurance
C. qualitative
D. quality control
E. kit
F. quantitative
G. reagent
H. proficiency testing
I. controls
J. accuracy
K. Levy-Jennings chart
L. medical office risk management
M. bar codes
N. reliability
O. standard deviation
P. precision
Q. internal control
R. external controls
S. mean

GOVERNMENT ACRONYMS WORKSHEET

As you write the words for each government acronym or abbreviation, notice its relationship to the various divisions of government and its effect on ambulatory laboratories.

Federal departments	HHS = Secretary of Health and Human Services				Department of Labor	
Divisions within the department	OCR = Office of Civil Rights	CMS = centers for medicare + medicaid services	FDA = food and drug administration	CDC = center of Disease Control	OSHA = occupational safety Health Administration	
Laws and/or regulations affecting laboratories	HIPAA: OCR enforces privacy standards	HIPAA: CMS enforces insurance portability		Infection control:	Infection control, blood:	Hazard communication standard
		CLIA: CMS administers the laboratory certifications	CLIA: FDA classifies laboratory test complexity	CDC recommends standard precautions for all infectious diseases	OSHA regulates BBPS = Blood-borne Pathogens standard	OSHA regulates chemical hazards
Additional acronyms and abbreviations	HIPAA = Health Insurance Portability and Accountability Act PHI = Protected health info.	CLIA = Clinical Lab. Improvement Amendments. QA = Quality assurance QC = quality contro	CoW = certificate of waiver. PPM = Provider-performed microscopy		PPE = personal protective equip. OPIM = other potentially infectious material PEP = post-exposure prophylaxis	MSDS = material safety data sheet HMIS = hazardous materials info. system. NFPA = National Fire Protection Association
Additional notes						

CLIA Government Regulations

20. What is the purpose of the Clinical Laboratory Improvement Amendment (CLIA 1988), and how does it benefit the patient?

    It protects the patients from inaccurate test results. CLIA is a regulation which the lab tests performed on specimens taken from the body for diagnose, prevention, or treatment of disease.

21. What are the three categories of testing under CLIA, and under which category is physician-performed microscopy listed?

    CLIA certificate of waiver, CLIA high and moderately complex labs, and CLIA Provider-Performed microscopy Procedures certificate. (PPMP)

22. Review Table 2-1 in the textbook, which lists most of the CLIA-waived tests available. Locate three tests in each category, and list their corresponding procedure codes on the chart:

Test Category	Physician Office Tests	Procedure Code (CPT; 5-digit code)
Hematology tests	Hemoglobin by copper sulfate	83026
	Blood count	85013
	Erythrocyte sedimentation rate.	85651
Blood chemistry tests	Cholestech LDX	82365 QW
	Hemo Cue B	82947 QW
	Blood chemistry Analyzer	80053 QW
Serology/immunology tests	Rapid wholeblood mononucleosis test	86308 QW
	Rapid whole blood test for Helicobacter pylori	86318 QW
	Orasure Oraquick rapid HIV-1 antibody test with whole blood	86701 QW
Microbiology tests (only two)	Quick Influenza A + B test	87804 QW
	Quick Streptococcus A test	87889 QW

23. From the provider-performed microscopy procedure in Table 2-2 in the textbook, write the procedure codes for each of the following:

    a. Wet mounts, including preparations of vaginal, cervical, or skin specimens ___Q0111___

    b. Urinalysis (microscopic only) ___81015___

    c. All potassium hydroxide preparations ___Q0112___

Chapter **2** **Regulations, Microscope Setup, and Quality Assurance**

24. Label the microscope, and perform the microscopic procedure at the end of the chapter.

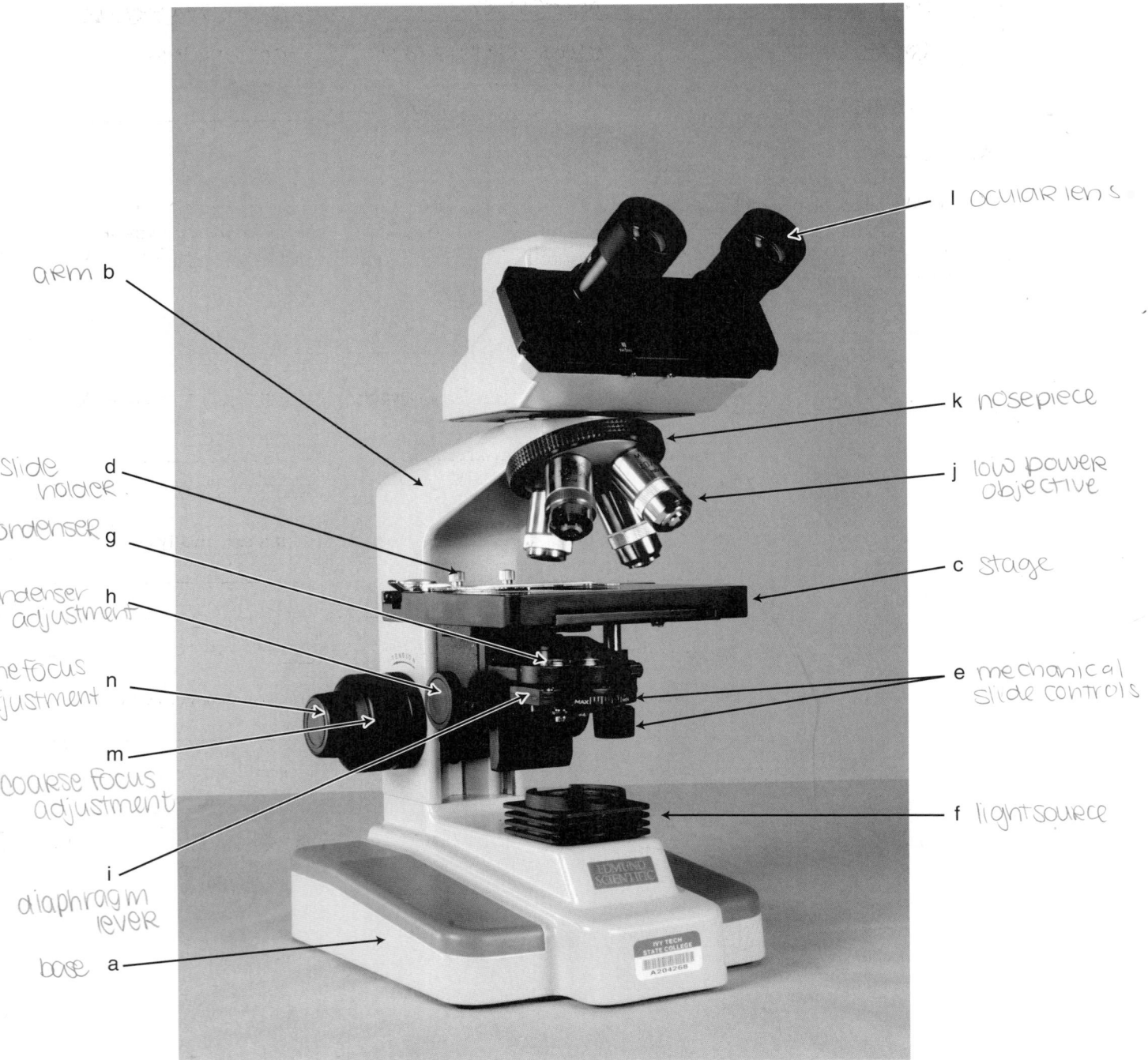

l ocular lens

arm b

k nosepiece

j low power objective

Slide holder d

condenser g

condenser adjustment h

c stage

fine focus adjustment n

e mechanical slide controls

m

coarse focus adjustment

f lightsource

i

diaphragm lever

base a

25. List three structures under each of the functional areas of the microscope.

Foundational	**Illuminating**	**Magnifying**
a. base	a. light source	a. objective lens
b. arm	b. condenser	b. focus adjustment knobs.
c. mechanical slide controls	c. diaphragm lever	c. ocular lens

FUNDAMENTAL CONCEPTS

Quality Control

26. Compare the 10 areas of good laboratory practices for certificate of waiver laboratories (Figure 2-2 in the textbook) with the flow chart of the three phases of laboratory testing requiring quality assessment (Table 2-3 in the textbook). Draw lines between the good laboratory practices numbers to divide the three phases of preanalytical, analytical, and postanalytical. Where should the lines be placed?

Between line 5+6

" " 6+7

27. Quality assurance oversees what areas of good laboratory practices? Quality control takes place during what areas of good laboratory practices? (All)

QA is overall process to aid in improving the reliability efficiency and quality of all lab test. QC is part of QA that takes place during the anallitical phase.

28. What is the difference between qualitative tests and quantitative tests, and how does it affect quality control?

Qualitative tests measure the presence or absence of a substance. (Results are either positive or negative) Quantitative tests produce results that have numerical values, where high and low values have diagnostic significance.

29. Explain the relationship of accuracy, precision, and reliability when plotting the results of standard controls.

Accuracy (correctness) occurs when control results consistently fall within central range. Precision occurs when results are clustered together on the target (produce the same test each time) Reliability is when both accuracy and precision are present.

30. Are laboratory personnel allowed to give an interested party a patient's test results? Why or why not? Base the answer on the Health Insurance Portability and Accountability Act (HIPAA) and risk management principles of avoiding financial and legal consequences.

No, because by HIPAA it is called protected health info, which means the lab results or any patient's information is confidential. We as laboratory personnel let the physician tell us the results and then let the patients know afterwards.

31. What is the single most important use of bar codes in the medical laboratory?

For positive patient and specimen identification throughout the entire testing process.

32. Plot 4 weeks of daily glucose control results on the four blank Levy-Jennings graphs. Mark the results for each day on the graph, and in the blank provided, identify whether the test system is experiencing a _trend_, a _shift_, a _random error_, or is _out of control_.
WEEK 1: day 1 = 103, day 2 = 100, day 3 = 98, day 4 = 112, day 5 = 105, day 6 = 99

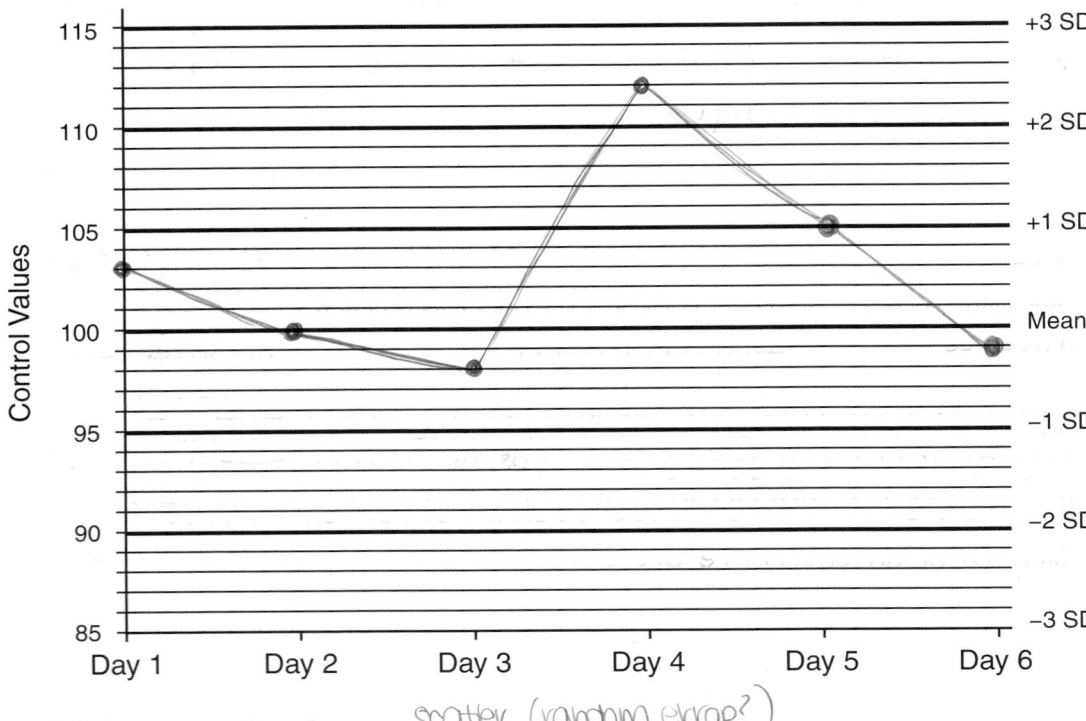

Week 1 glucose control results: _scatter (random error?)_

WEEK 2: day 1 = 94, day 2 = 92, day 3 = 93, day 4 = 108, day 5 = 109, day 6 = 107

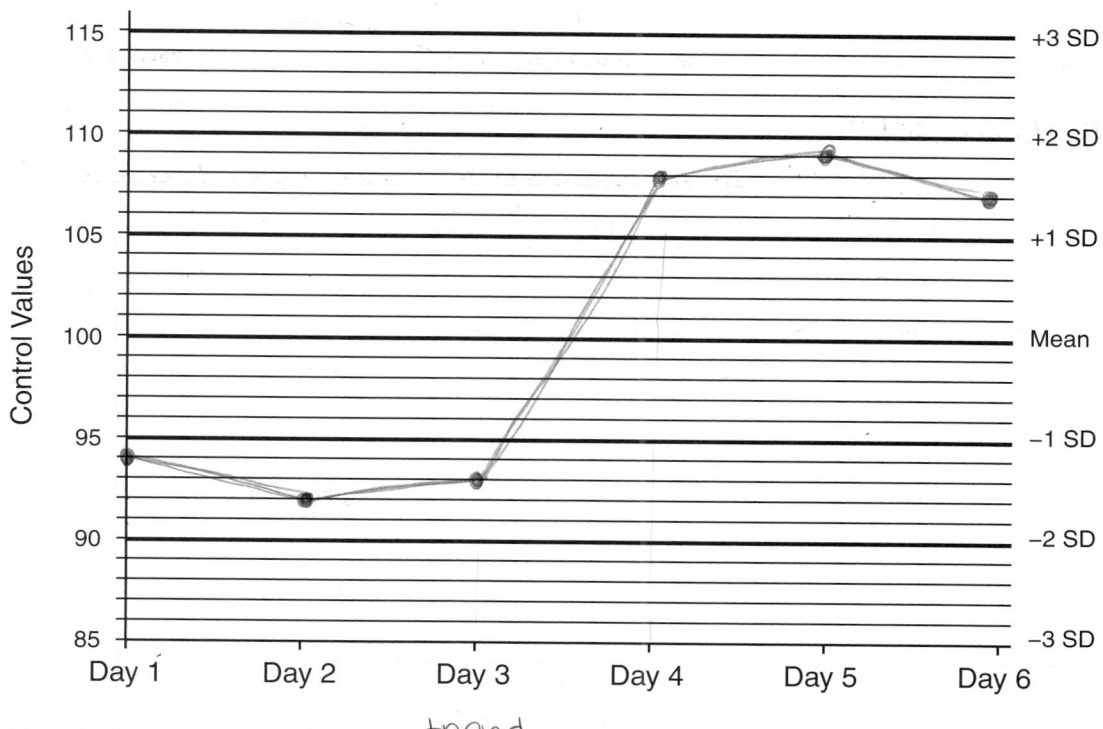

Week 2 glucose control results: _____ tRend _____

WEEK 3: day 1 = 90, day 2 = 95, day 3 = 100, day 4 = 105, day 5 = 108, day 6 = 110

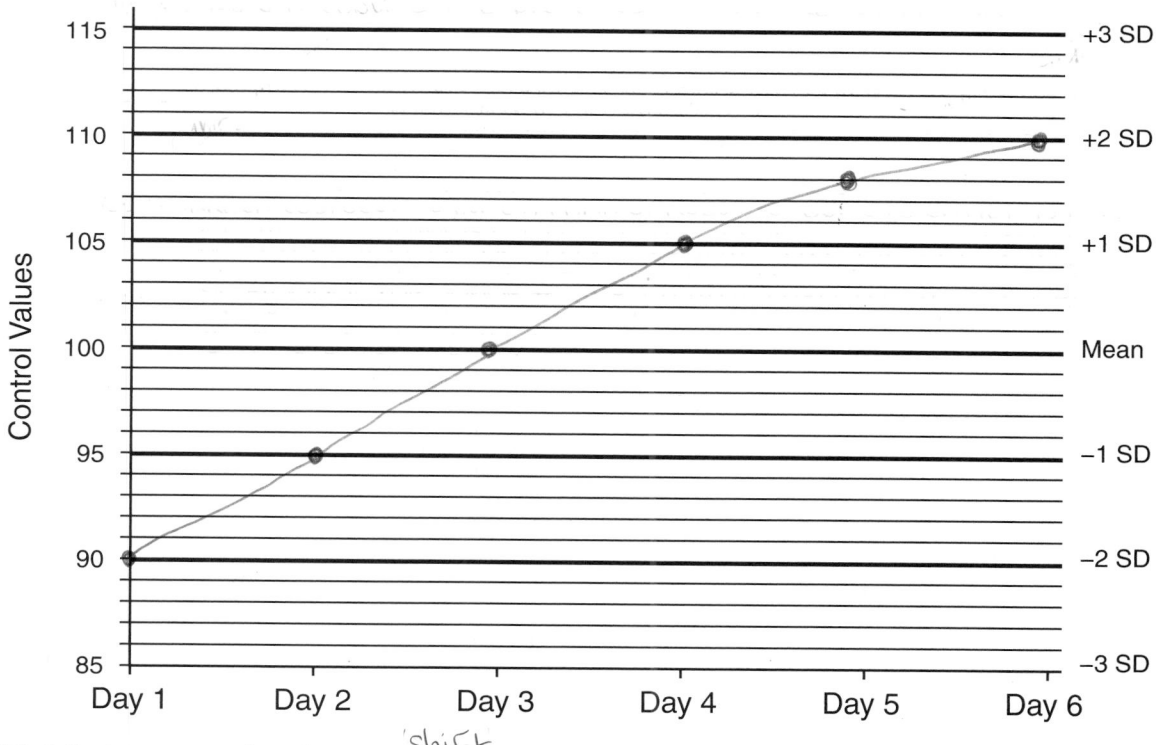

Week 3 glucose control results: _____ Shift _____

WEEK 4: day 1 = 100, day 2 = 103, day 3 = 98, day 4 = 112, day 5 = 115, day 6 = 113

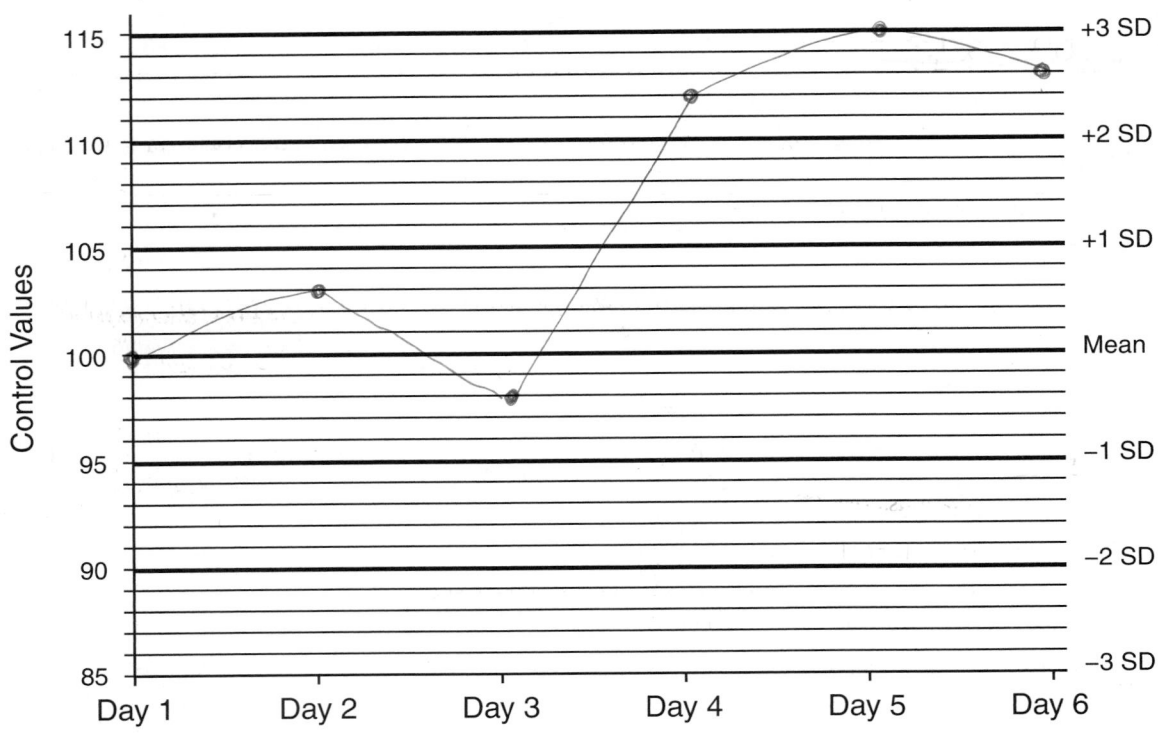

Week 4 glucose contol results: ___*out of control*___

3 Urinalysis

VOCABULARY REVIEW

Match the function with the correct anatomic term.

___f.___ 1. Functional unit of the kidney

___g.___ 2. Part of the nephron that contains the glomerulus and glomerular capsule

___b.___ 3. Structure in the renal corpuscle made up of tangled blood capillaries in which the hydrostatic pressure in the capillaries pushes substances through the capillary pores

___c.___ 4. Cup-shaped structure surrounding the glomerulus that collects the glomerular filtrate

___a.___ 5. Urethral opening through which urine is expelled

___h.___ 6. Slender, muscular tubes 10 to 12 inches long that carry the urine formed in the kidneys to the urinary bladder

___d.___ 7. Hollow, muscular organ that holds urine until it is expelled

___j.___ 8. Tube that carries urine outside the body

___i.___ 9. Located behind the peritoneal cavity

___e.___ 10. Parts of the nephron composed of proximal convoluted tubules, the nephron loop (loop of Henle), and distal convoluted tubules

A. urethral meatus
B. glomerulus
C. glomerular capsule
D. urinary bladder
E. renal tubules
F. nephron
G. renal corpuscle
H. ureters
I. retroperitoneal
J. urethra

Match each urinalysis term with the correct definition.

___p.___ 11. electrolyte

___w.___ 12. renal threshold level

___l.___ 13. oliguria

___t.___ 14. bilirubin

___i.___ 15. anuria

___e.___ 16. dysuria

___h.___ 17. nocturia

___s.___ 18. diuresis

___o.___ 19. porphyrin

___j.___ 20. glycosuria

___b.___ 21. reducing substances

___m.___ 22. ketonuria

A. Caused by treatment or diagnostic procedures
B. Substance that easily loses electrons
C. Intact red blood cells in the urine
D. Protein found in the urine of patients with multiple myeloma
E. Painful urination
F. Red cells breaking open and releasing hemoglobin
G. Expelling of urine, also referred to as voiding and urination
H. In urinalysis, the weight of urine compared with the weight of an equal volume of water; measures the amount of dissolved substances in urine
I. No urine flow
J. Sugars (especially glucose) in the urine
K. To break open
L. Decreased urine volume
M. Ketones in the urine
N. Excessive urination at night
O. Intermediate substance in the formation of heme (part of hemoglobin)
P. Element or compound that forms ions when dissolved and is able to conduct electricity

27

_____C_____ 23. hematuria
_____K_____ 24. lyse
_____F_____ 25. hemolysis
_____q_____ 26. proteinuria
_____U_____ 27. pyuria
_____a_____ 28. iatrogenic
_____R_____ 29. lipiduria
_____V_____ 30. casts
_____g_____ 31. micturition
_____X_____ 32. pH
_____h_____ 33. specific gravity
_____d_____ 34. Bence Jones protein

Q. Proteins in the urine
R. Lipids in the urine
S. Increase in the volume of urine output
T. Waste product from the breakdown of hemoglobin
U. White blood cells in the urine
V. Elements excreted in the urine in the shape of the renal tubules and ducts
W. Blood reabsorption limit of a substance and the point at which the substance is then excreted in the urine
X. Scale that measures the level of acidity or alkalinity of a solution

FUNDAMENTAL CONCEPTS

Anatomy of the Urinary System

35. Label the structures of the urinary system.

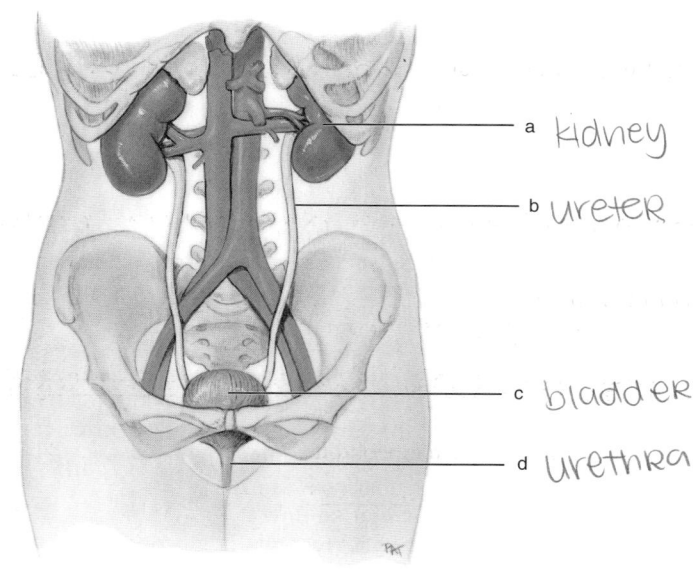

a Kidney
b ureter
c bladder
d urethra

36. Label the structures of the kidney.

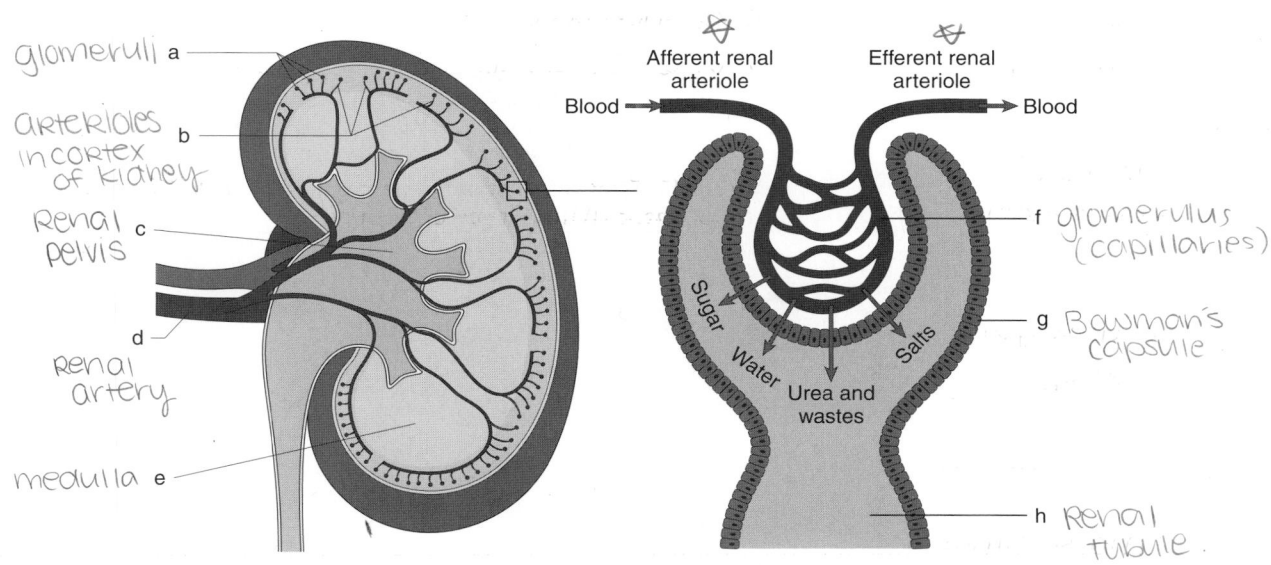

glomerulli a

arterioles b
in cortex
of kidney

Renal c
pelvis

d

Renal
artery

medulla e

Afferent renal
arteriole

Blood →

Efferent renal
arteriole

→ Blood

Sugar

Water

Salts

Urea and
wastes

f glomerullus
(capillaries)

g Bowman's
capsule

h Renal
tubule.

37. List three functions of the urinary system.

1. _Removes unwanted wastes._

2. _Stabilizes blood volume, acidity, and electrolytes._

3. _Secrets hormone erythropoietin and Renin._

38. Describe the location of the kidneys in the body.

Its located slightly above the waistline in the posterior wall of abdominal cavity, in a Retroperitoneal position.

39. List the functions of the nephron.

-filters waste substances from the blood.

-maintain the essential water and electrolyte balance of body.

40. Name the two structural components of the nephron.

Renal corpuscle and Renal tubules.

41. List and describe the components of the renal corpuscle.

Glomerulus is made up of tangled blood capillaries in which hydrostatic pressure in capillaries pushes substances through capillary pores.

Glomerular filtrate is collected in the Bowman's capsule and surrounds glomerulus.

42. Describe the three steps of urine formation.

Filtration (fluids + dissolved substances in blood are forced through pores of glom.)

Reabsorption (some substances that flow through renal tubules are needed by body cross back into blood by peritubular capillaries)

Secretion (substances are transported from peritubular blood capillaries into renal tubules)

29

43. Explain the term *renal threshold*.

When blood levels of a substance such as glucose reach a point at which no more can be reabsorbed, the substance is excreted in urine 160 – 180 mg/dL

44. Discuss the importance of a urinalysis.

Can be used for screening in a physical exam, assist the physician in diagnosis of pathological conditions, and determine the effectiveness of treatment.

45. Name the three parts of a urinalysis.

Physical analysis, chemical analysis, and microscopic analysis.

Urine Specimen Collection

46. Discuss the advantages of the first morning specimen.

It is most concentrated (dark yellow) which the urine becomes more dilute (lighter in color) as the day progresses and more fluid is consumed. Probability of detecting abnormalities increases and microscopic elements remain intact for longer period.

47. Give three general requirements for all types of urine collection methods.

Volume needed 25-50mL, container must be correctly labeled with patient's info, and outside of container should be disinfected.

48. Discuss the proper handling and discarding of urine specimens.

Gloves should be worn when recieving the specimen, labels should be correct, and requisition completed. Remove gloves and sanitize hands after urine is placed in testing area. Remaining urine flush in sink. Biohazard waste.

49. When educating a female patient about the steps involved in preparing for midstream clean catch urine, why must the patient understand the importance of wiping from front to back?

Because you will get microorganisms if wiping from back to front.

CLINICAL LABORATORY IMPROVEMENT AMENDMENT (CLIA)–WAIVED URINALYSIS TESTS

Physical Urinalysis

50. Name the tests that are part of the physical urinalysis.

    Observing the color, odor, appearance, ph, specific gravity.

51. List the terms used to describe the appearance of urine.

    Clear, hazy (slightly cloudy), cloudy, and turbid (very cloudy)

52. Give the range of normal color for urine.

    Straw colored (light yellow), to yellow, to amber (dark yellow).

53. In what condition can urine have a sweet or fruity odor?

    When there is a presence of ketones.

54. Discuss three abnormal urine colors and their causes.

    Yellow-brown - caused by bilirubin Resulting from excessive RBC destruction.
    Orange-yellow-caused by bilirubin or urobilinogen resulting from reduction in
    functioning of liver cells. Green -caused by biliverdin resulting from the
    oxidation of bilirubin.

55. Describe the relevance of the specific gravity test in the urinalysis.

    Measures the amount of particles that are dissolved in the urine,
    which indicates the ability of the kidneys to concentrate the urine.

Chemical Urinalysis

56. Discuss the difference between qualitative, quantitative, and semiquantitative testing.

    Qualitative is a method of the presence or absence of an analyte. Quant-
    itative have numerical value indicating the amount of substance present.
    semiquantitative determines the approximate quantity of analyte.

57. Label the urinalysis chemistry supplies (see Figure 3-10 in the textbook).

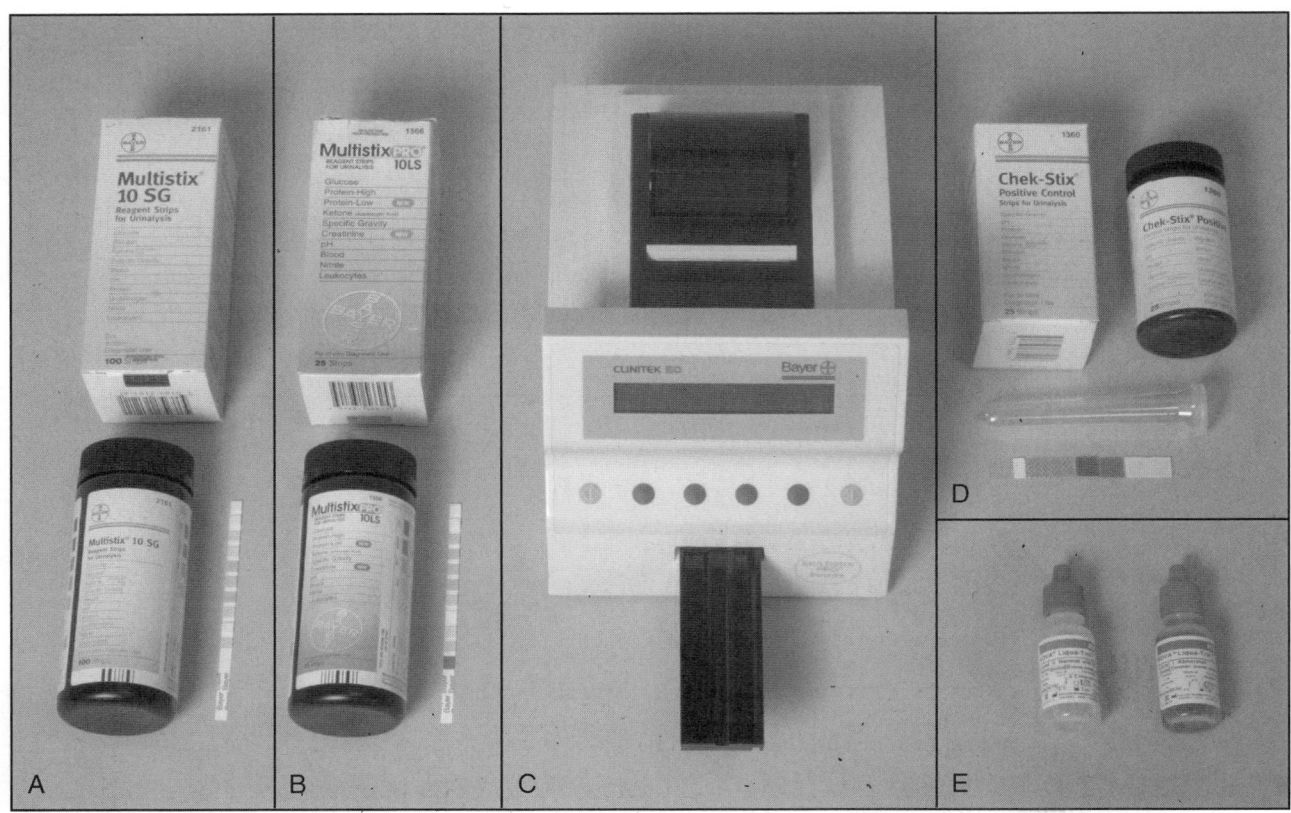

A ___Multi STIX 10SG___   B ___Multistix Pro___   C ___Clinitek___   D & E ___Chex Stix positive control strips___
   ___IOLS___   ___Kova normal + abnormal___
   ___controls.___

⭐ 58. Name the 10 urinalysis chemistry tests that are most frequently performed.

1. ___Specific gravity___   6. ___Urobilinogen___
2. ___pH___   7. ___Blood___
3. ___Glucose___   8. ___Protein___
4. ___Ketones___   9. ___Leukocytes___
5. ___Bilirubin___   10. ___Nitrites___

59. Discuss the reasons for the new method that tests for microalbumin.

It helps identify patient with nephropathy at a early stage.
It's critical for these condition, diabetes mellitus, hypertensive,
heart attack, stroke, and pregnancy.

60. List three conditions that may cause blood to be found in urine.

Kidney stones, tumors, menstrual period
, cystitis
urethritis

61. Explain why a first morning urine sample is recommended when testing for nitrites.

Because the urine must stay in the bladder for at least 4 to 6 hours to allow any bacteria that may be present sufficient time to convert nitrates to nitrites.

62. If the nitrite test is negative, could bacteria be present in the urine?   Yes

It doesn't mean that no bacterial infection is present. Some bacteria cannot convert nitrates to nitrite, or the urine didn't stay in bladder for 4 to 6 hrs.

63. Name a confirmatory test that can be performed when a urine sample is positive for the bilirubin test.

Ictotest can be performed.

64. Describe the Clinitek instrument, including its advantages and disadvantages.

The timing and color interpretation are consistent and do not vary among individual readers. A disadvantage is that if the urine contains a large amount of pigment, the machine cannot recognize this and will give false-positive results.

65. List three of the urinalysis chemistry reagent strip guidelines.

– must be read at a particular time
– must be kept tightly closed.
– keep the strips in a cool, dry place but not refrigerate.

66. Describe the quality control methods available for urinalysis chemistry testing. (Hint: see question 57.)

Use control strip containing synthetic ingredients. Results obtained must compared with manufacturer ranges. Must be logged in quality control quality record books.   pg 63

67. Circle the results that are abnormal compared with the urinalysis reference ranges. What is the probable cause for the abnormal urinalysis physical and chemical results, and what may the physician do next?
   • Dark yellow
   • Cloudy
   • Glucose–neg
   • Ketones–neg
   • Bilirubin–neg
   • Specific gravity 1.025
   • pH 7
   • Blood 2
   • Urobilinogen 0.2
   • Protein–mod
   • Nitrite–pos
   • Leukocyte–mod

Physician will order mid-stream catch.

68. Circle the results that are abnormal compared with the urinalysis reference ranges. What is the probable cause for the abnormal urinalysis chemical results?
    - (Glucose 2%)
    - Ketones–mod
    - Bilirubin–neg
    - Specific gravity 1.025
    - pH 6
    - Blood–neg
    - Urobilinogen 0.2
    - (Protein–trace)
    - Nitrite–neg
    - Leukocyte–neg

    uncontrolled diabetic

69. You just ran the Chek-Stix positive control and recorded the results shown. When looking at the expected results table for a positive control, circle the analyte that did **not** fall in its control range. Why do you suppose it did not record correctly? (Hint: Look at how the dipstick enters the urine specimen.)
    Glucose–neg
    Bilirubin–pos
    Ketones–pos
    Specific gravity 1.015
    Blood large
    pH 8.5
    Protein 100 mg/dL
    Urobilinogen 3 mg/dL
    Nitrate–pos
    Leukocytes–mod

Test	Expected Results with Bayer Reagent Strips and Tablets	
	Chek-Stix Positive Control	Chek-Stix Negative Control
Glucose	100-250 mg/dL	Negative
Bilirubin	Positive	Negative
Ketone	Positive	Negative
Specific gravity	1.000-1.015 (adjusted for pH)	1.010-1.025 (adjusted for pH)
Blood	Moderate, large	Negative
pH	≥8.0	6.0-7.0
Protein	Trace, 100 mg/dL (SI units: trace, 1.0 g/L)	Negative
Urobilinogen	≥2 mg/dL	0.2-1 mg/dL
Nitrite	Positive	Negative
Leukocytes	Trace, moderate	Negative
Microbumintest	Positive (by using 1:3 dilution of Chek-Stix positive control solution)	Negative
Acetest	Positive	Negative
Clinitest	250-750 mg/dL	Negative
Ictotest	Positive	Negative

70. For the standardized urinalysis Kova system for preparation of the microscopic examination, define the terms *sediment* and *supernatant,* and state which of these is used in the microscopic examination of urine.

    Sediment is material at the bottom of centrifuged tube of urine
    supernatant is liquid portion of urine on top of spun sediment.

71. List conditions in which *Candida albicans* (yeast) may be found in the urine.

    women with vaginal infection, patient with diabetes mellitus, and in
    immuno comprised patients.

72. Name the four factors that can lead to cast formation. decrease urine form, increase plasma protein

    Protein aggregates into individual protein fibrils that attach to renal tubule cells.
    Protein fibrils interweave, forming a loose fibrils network that becomes solid.
    Urinary components may attach to the solid structure.
    Protein fibril structure detaches from the epithelial cells and is excreted as
    cast.

73. Name the crystals that resemble envelopes (with an X appearance).

    Calcium oxalate crystals

74. What part of the microscopic urinalysis can be performed by a medical assistant?

    Preparing microscopic slide.

75. Match the pictures of urine cells, casts, and crystals with their microscopic drawings. (See Figures 3-14 through 3-37 on pages 76 to 80 in your textbook.)

Cells

Use these terms to identify the following illustrations: Red blood cells (RBCs) on high power, squamous epithelial cells on high power, transitional epithelial cells on high power, white blood cells (WBCs) on high power.

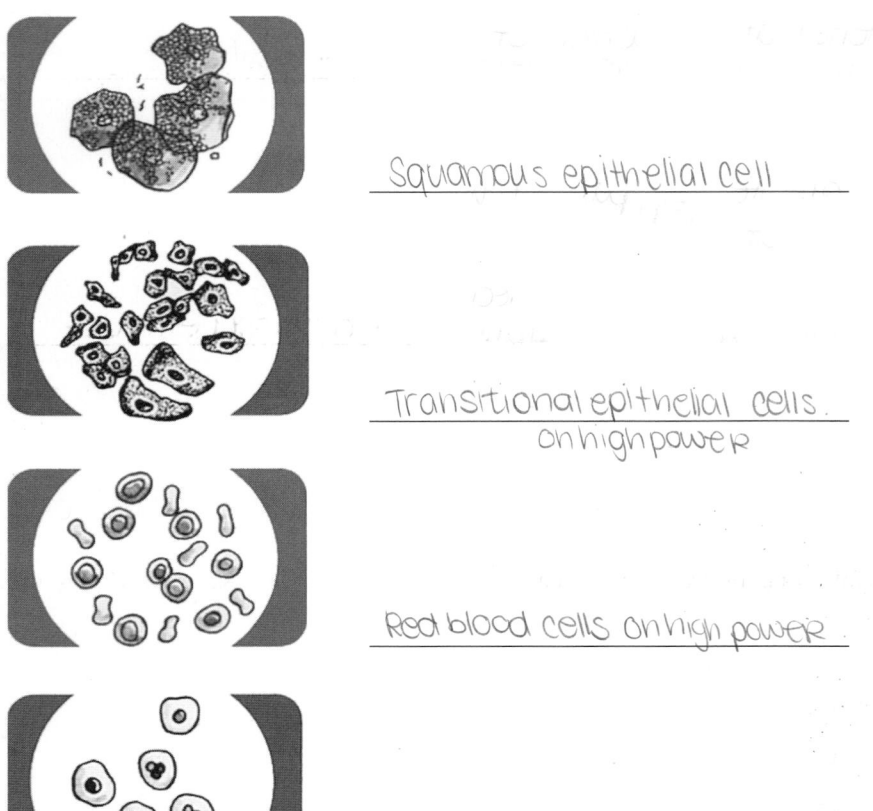

Squamous epithelial cell

Transitional epithelial cells. on high power

Red blood cells on high power

White blood cells on high power

Casts

Use these terms to identify the following illustrations: granular casts, hyaline casts, RBC casts, WBC casts.

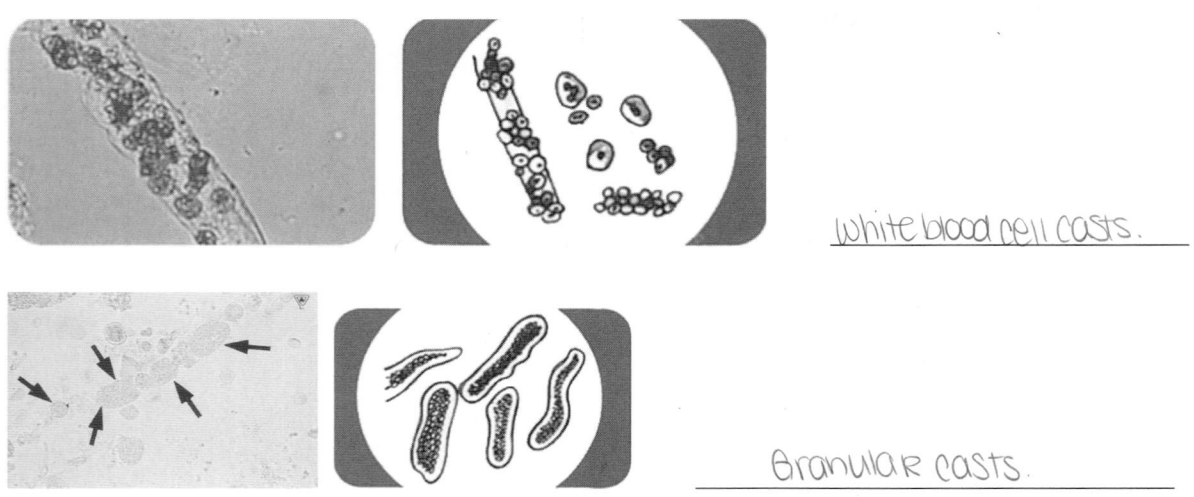

White blood cell casts.

Granular casts.

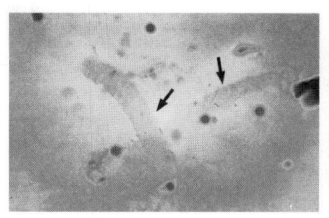 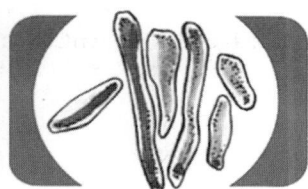

Hyaline casts

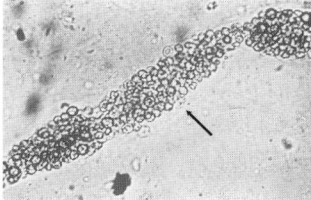 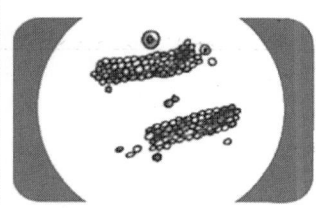

Red blood cell casts.

Crystals and Other Forms

Use these terms to identify the following illustrations: calcium oxalate crystals, *Trichomonas vaginalis*, triple phosphate crystals, yeast.

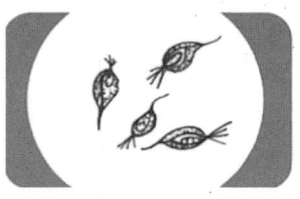

Trichomonas vaginalis

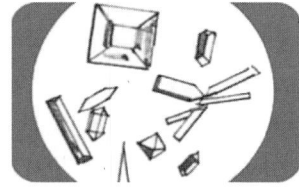

Triple phosphate crystals.

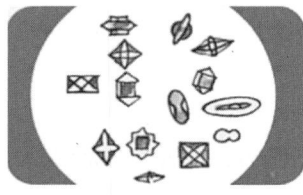

Calcium oxalate crystals

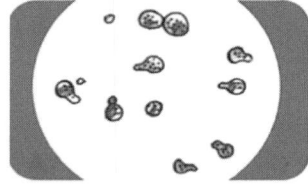

Yeast in urine.

38

Chapter **3** **Urinalysis**

Procedure 3-1: Instructing Patients How to Collect a Clean-Catch Urine Specimen—Female

Person evaluated _____ Date_____

Evaluated by _____ Score_____

Outcome goal	Instruct a female patient regarding the correct procedure for midstream clean catch specimen
Conditions	Given the following: - Sterile urine collection container and label - Antiseptic towelettes
Standards	Required time = 15 minutes Performance time = _____

Evaluation Rubric Codes:
S = Satisfactory, meets standard   **U** = Unsatisfactory, fails to meet standard

Total possible points = _____   Points earned = _____

NOTE: Steps marked with an asterisk (*) are critical to achieve required competency.

Preparation	Scores	
	S	U
1. Washed hands and gathered the appropriate equipment.		
2. Greeted and identified the patient.		

Procedure	Scores	
	S	U
3. Instructed patient to sanitize her hands and remove underwear.		
4. Instructed patient to spread apart the labia to expose the urinary opening.		
- Patient told to keep this area spread apart with the nondominant hand during the entire cleaning procedure.		
5. Instructed patient to take one antiseptic towelette and clean one side of the urinary opening from front to back, stressing the importance of the direction.		
- Patient told that cleaning in this direction will prevent anal organisms from being spread to the urinary opening.		
6. Instructed patient to take another antiseptic towelette and clean other side of the urinary opening from front to back, stressing the importance of the direction.		
7. Instructed patient using a third antiseptic towelette to wipe from front to back directly across the urinary opening, stressing the importance of the direction.		
8. Instructed patient to continue to keep labia spread apart and to urinate a small amount (one third of bladder volume) into the toilet, being careful not to touch the inside of the sterile container.		
- Patient told that the reason for a small amount urinated in the toilet is to flush away microorganisms that may be around the urinary opening.		

	Scores	
	S	U
9. Instructed patient to collect the second part of the urine sample into the sterile container.		
- Student was able to state that this would collect the midstream portion of the urine specimen.		
10. Instructed patient to urinate the last portion of the urine into the toilet.		
11. Instructed patient to dry the area with a tissue.		
12. Instructed the patient on the correct procedure after the specimen has been collected.		
- Instructed the patient to carefully cap the specimen.		
- Instructed patient to place specimen in a certain area after collected in an office setting or to refrigerate if collected at home.		

	Scores	
Follow-up	S	U
13. After receiving the specimen from the patient, the sample was labeled correctly, and the requisition was completed if required.		
14. Washed hands.		
*15. Procedure was charted correctly.		
- Charted that female patient was given instructions for midstream clean catch urine collection.		
- Charted reception of specimen from patient.		
Total Points per Column		

Patient Chart Entry: (Include when, what, how, why, any additional information, and the signature of the person charting.)

_____

_____

_____

Procedure 3-1: Instructing Patients How to Collect a Clean-Catch Urine Specimen—Male

Person evaluated _____   Date_____

Evaluated by _____   Score_____

Outcome goal	Instruct a male patient in the correct procedure for midstream clean catch specimen
Conditions	Given: - Sterile urine collection container and label - Antiseptic towelettes
Standards	Required time = 15 minutes Performance time = _____
Evaluation Rubric Codes: **S** = Satisfactory, meets standard **U** = Unsatisfactory, fails to meet standard Total possible points = _____ Points earned = _____	
NOTE: Steps marked with an asterisk (*) are critical to achieve required competency.	

Preparation	Scores	
	S	**U**
1. Washed hands and gathered the appropriate equipment.		
2. Greeted and identified the patient.		

Procedure	Scores	
	S	**U**
3. Instructed patient to sanitize his hands and remove underwear.		
4. If patient is uncircumcised, instructed the patient to retract the foreskin and hold it back during the entire procedure.		
5. Instructed the patient to clean the area around the penis opening by starting at the tip of the penis and cleaning downward, using a separate antiseptic towelette for each side.		
6. Instructed patient to use a third antiseptic towelette to clean across the opening.		
*7. Instructed patient to urinate a small amount (one third of bladder volume) into the toilet, being careful not to touch the inside of the sterile container.		
- Patient told that the reason for a small amount urinated in the toilet is to flush away microorganisms that may be around the urinary opening.		
8. Instructed patient to collect the second part of the urine sample into the sterile container.		
- Student was able to state that this would collect the midstream portion of the urine specimen.		
9. Instructed patient to urinate the last portion of the urine into the toilet.		
10. Instructed patient to dry the area with a tissue if needed.		

Follow-up	Scores	
	S	**U**
11. Instructed the patient on the correct procedure after the specimen has been collected.		
- Instructed the patient to carefully cap the specimen.		
- Instructed patient to place specimen in a certain area after collected in an office setting or to refrigerate if collected at home.		
12. After receiving the specimen from the patient, the sample was labeled correctly and the requisition was completed if required.		
13. Washed hands.		
*14. Charted procedure correctly.		
- Charted that male patient was given instructions for midstream clean catch urine collection.		
- Charted reception of specimen from patient.		
Total Points per Column		

Patient Chart Entry: (Include when, what, how, why, any additional information, and the signature of the person charting.)

_____

_____

_____

Procedure 3-2: Instructing Patients How to Collect a 24-Hour Urine Specimen

Person evaluated _____   Date_____

Evaluated by _____   Score_____

Outcome goal	To educate the patient on the correct instructions for collection of a 24-hour urine specimen
Conditions	Given: - Large urine container - Instructions sheet - Requisition
Standards	Required time = 15 minutes Performance time = _____

Evaluation Rubric Codes:
S = Satisfactory, meets standard   **U** = Unsatisfactory, fails to meet standard

Total possible points = _____   Points earned = _____

NOTE: Steps marked with an asterisk (*) are critical to achieve required competency.

Preparation	Scores	
	S	U
1. Washed hands and gathered the appropriate equipment.		
2. Greeted and identified the patient.		

Procedure	Scores	
	S	U
3. Instructed patient when arising on the first day of the 24-hour collection procedure to empty bladder into the toilet.		
- Instructed patient to record this time.		
4. Instructed the patient that all urine for 24 hours after that first voided specimen must be voided directly into the collection container.		
- Informed the patient to be sure to screw the lid on tightly each time and keep the container refrigerated.		
- Informed the patient that if at any time during the procedure some urine is not collected, the test will need to start again. Gave examples of this.		
5. Instructed the patient that on the second morning of the 24-hour period the patient must arise at the same time as the first day and urinate directly into the container, keeping this sample.		
- Patient was instructed that the first morning specimen on the second day 24-hour period is the last sample collected and is the completion of the collection procedure.		
6. Instructed the patient that on the day the procedure is completed, the container must be returned to the physician's office or to the laboratory.		

Follow-up	Scores	
	S	U
7. After the patient completed the procedure and returned the container, the patient was asked if any problems occurred during the collection procedure.		
8. Completed a laboratory requisition form for test ordered.		
9. Prepared the specimen to be transported to the laboratory that will perform the testing.		
*10. Charted the instructions and equipment supplied to the patient.		
- When patient returned with specimen, charted that the specimen was sent to the laboratory, documenting all necessary information concerning the specimen.		
Total Points per Column		

Patient Chart Entry: (Include when, what, how, why, any additional information, and the signature of the person charting.)

_____

_____

_____

Procedure 3-5: Clinitest Procedure for Reducing Substances Such as Sugars in the Urine

Person evaluated _____ Date_____

Evaluated by _____ Score_____

Outcome goal	Perform a Clinitest test on an unknown sample
Conditions	Given: - Clinitest bottle of tablets - Clinitest tube - Tube of water with pipette - Urine sample with pipette - Clinitest reference chart
Standards	Required time = 5 minutes Performance time = _____
Evaluation Rubric Codes: **S** = Satisfactory, meets standard	**U** = Unsatisfactory, fails to meet standard
Total possible points = _____	Points earned = _____
NOTE: Steps marked with an asterisk (*) are critical to achieve required competency	

Preparation: Preanalytical Phase	Scores	
	S	**U**
A. Test information		
- Kit or instrument method: **Clinitest**		
- Manufacturer: **Bayer Corporation**		
- Proper storage (e.g., temperature, light): **room temperature with the lid tightly sealed; protect tablets from light, heat, and moisture**		
- Lot number of kit: _____		
- Expiration date: _____		
- Package insert available: _____ yes _____ no		
B. Specimen information		
- Labeled urine specimen in clean container		
- Amount: **2 or 5 drops (according to directions)**		
C. Personal protective equipment: **gloves, sharps, and biohazard**		

Procedure: Analytical Phase	Scores	
	S	U
D. Performed/observed quality control		
1. Semiquantitative testing controls		
- Control levels: Normal _____ Abnormal _____		
E. Performed patient test	S	U
1. Added 5 drops of urine to 10 drops of water in a Clinitest tube.		
2. Tapped the Clinitest tablet into the tube, which was placed in a rack because the boiling reaction that occurs is very hot.		
3. During the boiling reaction, the tube was observed for any color change.		
- The boiling reaction should be observed for the "pass through effect," which results with color change occurring during the reaction and appears negative when the reaction is completed and results are determined.		
4. Shook the tube 15 seconds after the boiling had stopped to mix the contents.		
5. Compared color of the reaction with the Clinitest chart for the 5-drop method and recorded the results.		

*Accurate Results _____   Instructor Confirmation _____

Follow-up: Postanalytical Phase	Scores	
	S	U
*F. Proper documentation_____		
1. On control log: _____ yes _____ no		
2. On patient log: _____ yes _____ no		
3. Documentation on patient chart (see below).		
4. Identified critical values and took appropriate steps to notify physician. Expected values for analyte: **negative**		
G. Proper disposal and disinfection		
1. Disposed all other regulated medical waste into biohazard bags.		
2. Disinfected test area and instruments according to OSHA guidelines.		
3. Sanitized hands after removing gloves.		
Total Points per Column		

Patient Name: _____

Patient Chart Entry: (Include when, how, what, why, any additional information, and the signature of the person charting.)

_____

_____

_____

Procedure 3-6: Procedure for the Preparation and the Microscopic Examination of Urine

Person evaluated _____   Date_____

Evaluated by _____   Score_____

Outcome goal	To prepare a microscopic urinalysis slide, focus the slide on the microscope, and state the elements that can be found under low and high power
Conditions	Given: - Gloves - Urine specimen - Kova equipment: cap, pipette - Sternheimer-Malbin stain - Test tube - Centrifuge - Microscope
Standards	Required time = 5 minutes Performance time = _____

Evaluation Rubric Codes:
S = Satisfactory, meets standard   **U** = Unsatisfactory, fails to meet standard

Total possible points = _____   Points earned = _____

NOTE: Steps marked with an asterisk (*) are critical to achieve required competency.

Preparation	Scores	
	S	U
1. Washed hands, applied gloves, and gathered the appropriate equipment.		
2. Mixed the correctly identified room temperature urine specimen.		
3. Poured the urine sample to the "12 mark" in a urine centrifuge tube and capped the tube.		

Procedure	Scores	
	S	U
4. Centrifuged the tube for 5 minutes at 1500 rpm.		
- Stated the definition of sediment and supernatant.		
5. Carefully removed the spun tube from the centrifuge and removed the cap.		
6. Carefully placed the Kova pipette into the bottom of the tube.		
- Hooked the clip on the top of the pipette over the outside of the tube.		
7. Placed index finger on tip of the pipette and decanted off the supernatant by inverting the tube.		
- Stated the approximate amount of sediment that remained in the tube.		

	S	U
8. Removed the pipette from the tube, added a drop of stain, and reinserted the pipette, squeezing gently to mix the urine sediment and stain.		
- Stated the purpose of using the stain.		
9. Correctly transferred a drop of the urine sediment to a well in a Kova slide.		
- Did not overfill or underfill the well.		
10. Allowed the Kova slide to sit for 1 minute.		
- Stated why the slide should sit.		
11. Stated who is qualified to perform a urine microscopic examination.		
12. Demonstrated the ability to focus a slide on the microscope.		
- Focused first with low power with the course adjustment.		
- Was able to fine focus with the fine adjustment knob.		
*13. Stated what elements are observed under low power.		
*14. Stated what elements are observed under high power.		

*Accurate Results _____   Instructor Confirmation _____

Follow-up: Postanalytical Phase	Scores	
	S	U
15. Demonstrated the proper procedure for cleaning, carrying, and storing the microscope.		
16. Correctly discarded the equipment in the appropriate containers.		
- Discarded the urine specimen in the appropriate manner.		
17. Removed and discarded gloves in the appropriate biohazard containers.		
18. Sanitized hands.		
19. Demonstrated an understanding of the process for calculating a urinalysis microscopic examination.		
Total Points per Column		

Patient Chart Entry: (Include when, what, how, why, any additional information, and the signature of the person charting.)

_____

_____

_____

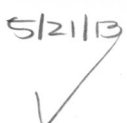

5/21/13

4 Blood Collection

VOCABULARY REVIEW

Match each term with the correct definition.

<u>e.</u> 1. cyanotic
<u>f.</u> 2. edema
<u>o.</u> 3. syncope
<u>j.</u> 4. petechiae
<u>L.</u> 5. plasma
<u>N.</u> 6. veins
<u>a.</u> 7. antecubital space
<u>d.</u> 8. capillary action
<u>b.</u> 9. arteries
<u>g.</u> 10. hematoma
<u>h.</u> 11. interstitial fluid
<u>k.</u> 12. phlebotomy
<u>m.</u> 13. serum
<u>i.</u> 14. osteomyelitis
<u>c.</u> 15. capillaries
<u>q.</u> 16. buffy coat
<u>R.</u> 17. humors
<u>V.</u> 18. evacuate
<u>P.</u> 19. palpating
<u>t.</u> 20. hemoconcentration
<u>S.</u> 21. lumen
<u>u.</u> 22. microcollection

A. Area in front of the elbow
B. Blood vessels that carry blood away from the heart
C. Microscopic blood vessels that contain a mixture of arterial and venous blood
D. Process by which blood flows freely into a capillary tube in microcollection procedures
E. Condition in which the skin and mucous membranes are blue; caused by an oxygen deficiency
F. Abnormal collection of fluid in interstitial spaces
G. Tumor or swelling of blood in the tissues (resulting in bruising during blood collection procedures)
H. All the fluid, except blood, found in the space between tissues; also referred to as tissue fluid
I. Inflammation of the bone caused by bacterial infection
J. Tiny purple or red skin spots caused by small amounts of blood under the skin; found in those with coagulation problems; can lead to excessive bleeding during phlebotomy procedures
K. Blood collection; derived from the Greek words *phlebo*, meaning vein, and *tomy*, meaning to cut
L. Liquid part of whole blood
M. Liquid part obtained when blood is clotted; lacks the clotting factors
N. Blood vessels that carry blood toward the heart
O. Fainting
P. Gently touching and pressing down on an area to feel texture, size, and consistency
Q. Narrow middle layer of white blood cells and platelets in a centrifuged whole blood specimen
R. Fluid or semifluid substances found in the body
S. Inner tubular space of a needle, vessel, or tube
T. Condition in which blood concentration of large molecules such as proteins, cells, and coagulation factors increases
U. Collecting a small amount of blood
V. Removing air to produce a vacuum

FUNDAMENTAL CONCEPTS

23. Explain the differences between arteries, arterioles, capillaries, venules, and veins.

Arteries carry blood away from heart. Veins carry blood to the heart. Arterioles are small arteries and venules are small veins. Capillaries are microscopic blood vessels where exchange of materials with tissues takes place and it carry a mixture of arterial and venous blood.

57

24. Determine if the following substances are higher in the capillary or venous blood.

   a. Hemoglobin ___capillary___

   b. Total protein ___venous blood___

   c. Potassium ___venous blood___

   d. Glucose ___capillary___

   e. Calcium ___venous blood___

25. Describe the difference in the "feel" between an artery and a vein.

   ___Veins feel spongy, and arteries feel more elastic and have a pulse.___

26. Draw a diagram of the most common veins in the antecubital area used for phlebotomy.

27. List the seven items that must be on a requisition.

   a. ___Patient's name___

   b. ___Patient's id number___

   c. ___Patient's date of birth___

   d. ___Name of test ordered___

   e. ___Name of physician ordering test___

   f. ___Timing of test___

   g. ___Insurance or billing info.___

28. What is the most critical error that a phlebotomist can make?

   ___Misidentification of patient___

29. Describe the three-way match for patient identification.

   ___Matching the patient's name and date of birth with test requisition,___
   ___plus one more type of id such as drivers license, hospital id #.___

30. Explain the proper way to determine a patient's name.

Ask, "What's your name" or "Spell your name."

31. Describe and explain the correct positions of a patient when performing phlebotomy.

Have the patient sit in a chair with armrest

BLOOD COLLECTION PROCEDURES

Capillary Puncture

32. Describe the composition of capillary blood.

It's not the same as that of venous blood. Because capillaries are a bridge between arteries and veins, a skin puncture draws blood from arterioles, venules, and capillaries as well as interstitual fluid.

33. Label the capillary puncture supplies.

gloves   gauze   alcohol wipes

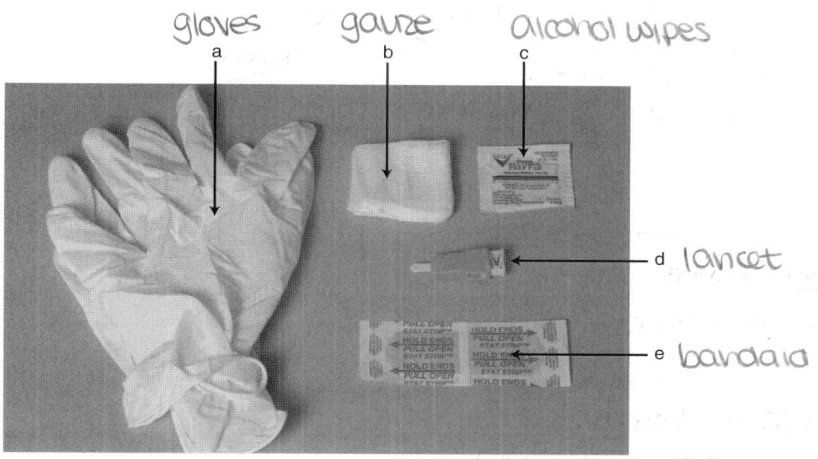

a   b   c

d _lancet_

e _bandaid_

34. List three situations when capillary blood may be used and three situations when this method should not be used.

Be used
① _When only small amount of blood is needed_
② _With children, because of risks of venipuncture_
③ _With cancer, geriatric, or obese patients, whose blood can be difficult_

NOT
① _If test requires large amount of blood._
② _If patient has poor peripheral circulation._
③ _If interstitial fluid could dilute the test, causing inaccurate results._

35. What is the recommended capillary puncture depth for newborns and infants? Explain why.

It should not exceed 2mm to prevent infection caused by puncturing a bone.

36. List two types of tubes that can be used to collect the blood from capillary punctures. (Hint: see Figure 4-6C and D in the textbook.)

· Capillary tubes and microcollection tubes microtainers with

37. List and explain the recommended order of collecting the various colored microtainers from a capillary puncture.

Lavender tubes containing EDTA, used for hematology tests. Other tubes containing anticoagulation additives (green-topped tubes) with anticoagulant heparin and followed by 2 blue and then grey. Nonadditive tubes (red-topped tubes that contain no anticoagulants, clot accelerators, or gels.

38. Describe the appropriate capillary puncture collection sites for adults and children and then for newborns and infants.

Adults and children: middle or ring finger.

Infants and newborns: medial or lateral plantar surface of the heel.

39. Why is the first drop of blood wiped away in a capillary puncture?

Because it contains tissue fluid that could dilute the sample.

40. Discuss the effects if alcohol is not allowed to dry when performing blood collection.

It may cause hemolysis, contaminate glucose determinations, or prevent drops of blood from forming.

41. What will squeezing the puncture site do to the test results?

Squeezing can cause the blood sample to be contaminated with tissue fluid.

42. Describe what to do if the blood stops flowing and not enough blood was obtained.

Entire procedure should be repeated at a new site with a new sterile puncture device.

43. Describe phenylketonuria (PKU).

It's a screening for newborns which determines if newborn lacks the enzymes needed for certain metabolic reactions.

44. Describe the neonatal screening collection procedure.

WARM the heel and a capillary puncture is done on lateral of heel. Wipe away first drop of blood then collect the blood in microtainer or screening card. Apply drop of blood to each circle. All circles must be filled. Allow to dry in horizontal position for 3 mins. Mail the forms to testing center.

45. Discuss the infant age parameters for testing for PKU.

24 hrs - 72 hrs after birth. If screening is done before child is 24 hrs old, it must be repeated before the child is 14 days old.

46. In the following case study steps, write **C** if the technique is correct or **I** if the technique is incorrect; explain why in the space provided.
A medical assistant performs a capillary puncture on an adult.

___C___ 1. The medical assistant washes his or her hands and puts on gloves.

___C___ 2. The site that is chosen is the lateral part of the fingertip (slightly to the side of center) of the middle finger.

___I___ 3. The site is cleaned with 30% alcohol.
70% aqueous solution of isopropyl alcohol.

___I___ 4. The puncture is made before the site is dry.
After the site is dry.

___I___ 5. The puncture is made parallel to the whorls of the fingerprint.
perpendicular.

47. In the following scenario about a capillary puncture, circle the incorrect techniques. In the space provided, explain the repercussions that could occur from using the incorrect method.

A capillary puncture is performed on the central area of the heel of a newborn infant's foot. The area is cleaned with 70% alcohol, and before it has dried, a puncture is made with a lancet to a depth of 3 mm. Immediately after the puncture, the blood is collected in a capillary tube by squeezing the puncture site. After all the blood has been obtained, pressure is applied to the puncture site, and an adhesive bandage is applied.

- lateral area of the infant's heel. - Wait until it's dried. cause of hemolysis. - depth is 2mm to avoid infection. - massage slightly to avoid bruising.

48. Explain the difference between serum and plasma, and describe how each is obtained.

Serum is liquid part obtained when blood is clotted. Plasma is liquid part of whole blood.

✗ test

49. Label the parts of the Vacutainer system.

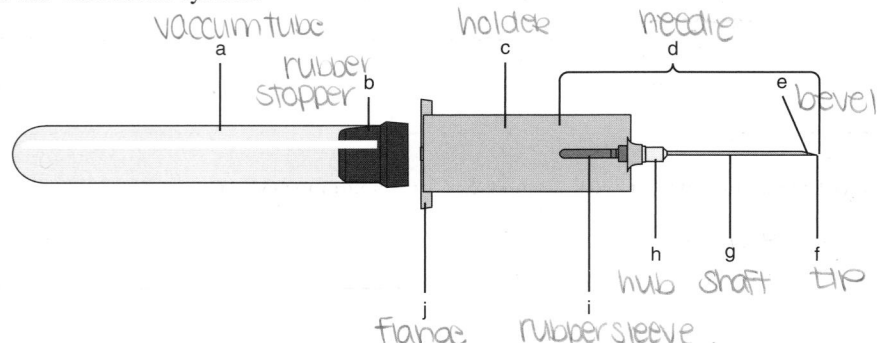

vaccum tube a
rubber stopper b
holder c
needle d
bevel e
hub h
shaft g
tip f
flange j
rubber sleeve i

50. Place the following tubes in the correct order of draw, and name the anticoagulant or additive in each: green, gray, red, lavender.

a. ___Red___ ; No anticoagulant / has clot activator.
b. ___green___ ; heparin anticoagulant.
c. ___lavender___ ; EDTA
d. ___gray___ ; potassium oxalate / sodium fluoride anticoagulant.

51. Describe how a gel separator tube functions.

It forms a barrier between the cells and the liquid to stop further interaction between these layers.

52. Describe the function of the tourniquet. Include the appropriate distance from the puncture site a tourniquet should be placed and the recommended time it should be on the arm.

It's used to make the vein more prominent and easier to puncture. It is a 1 inch wide and 15 - 18 inches long and should be placed 3 to 4 inches above venipuncture site.

53. Discuss the criteria for determining whether a tourniquet is on correctly.

It should be tight enough to restrict venous flow but not so tight that it stops arterial flow.

54. List the assets and limitations of the topical anesthetic EMLA.

Its a topical cream that is a mixture of lidocaine and prilocaine. Limitations are costs, the need to wait 60 mins, and need to repeat anesthetizing procedure.

55. Why should the tourniquet be released before removing the needle?

So the blood don't squirt out everywhere.

56. Why does the needle need to be held steady during the venipuncture procedure?

It is more comfortable for the patient.

57. Name the three methods that can be used to obtain blood from a vein.

Vacuum tube method

Syringe method

Butterfly method

58. What are the most frequently used needle gauges for the Vacutainer system?

20 to 22 gauges

59. List the advantages of using the Vacutainer method.

· It is smoother and less painful puncture, tubes automatically fills.

60. Explain when a butterfly and syringe method would be used.

It is used when veins are thin or might collapse.

61. Describe the safety steps of discarding the needle after removing it from the arm with the Vacutainer method.

Activate the needle safety device and discard the entire Vacutainer device in a biohazard sharps container.

62. List three conditions that could cause a hematoma.

needle goes through the vein

needle is only partially in the vein.

Insufficient pressure is applied to the puncture site after procedure is completed.

63. Describe the recommended procedure for transferring blood from a syringe into vacuum tubes.

must be transferred quickly so the blood doesn't clot. Transfer the blood from syringe to vacuum tubes with safety transfer device.

64. Describe the procedure for determining the appropriate vein for venipuncture.

Begin one side of antecubital space and palpate across to the other side with the index finger. The vein will feel spongy.

65. Identify and describe the function of each part of the syringe system.

Syringe consists of barrel and plunger.

Syringe needle (hypodermic needle) has a shaft and hub.

66. Label the parts of the syringe.

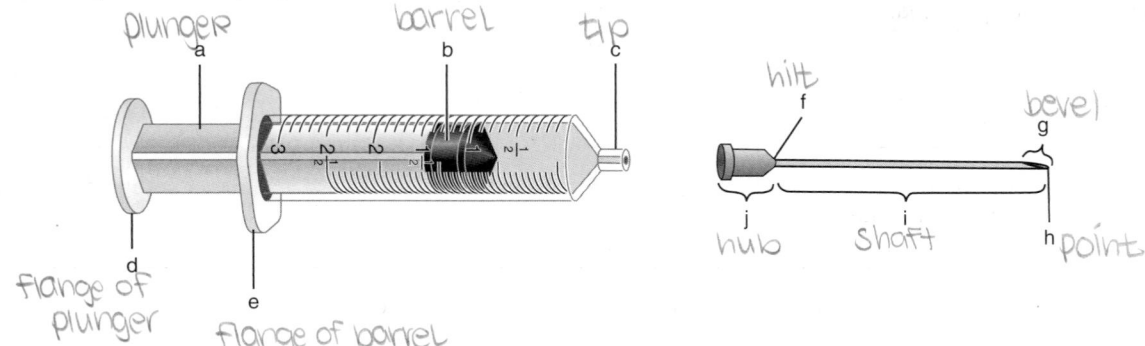

plunger a
barrel b
tip c
flange of plunger d
e flange of barrel
hilt f
bevel g
j hub
i shaft
h point

67. Identify and describe the function of each of the components of the butterfly system, including use of the Luer Adapter/Vacutainer method and the syringe method.

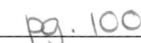 pg. 100

68. Label the supplies needed for the butterfly system.

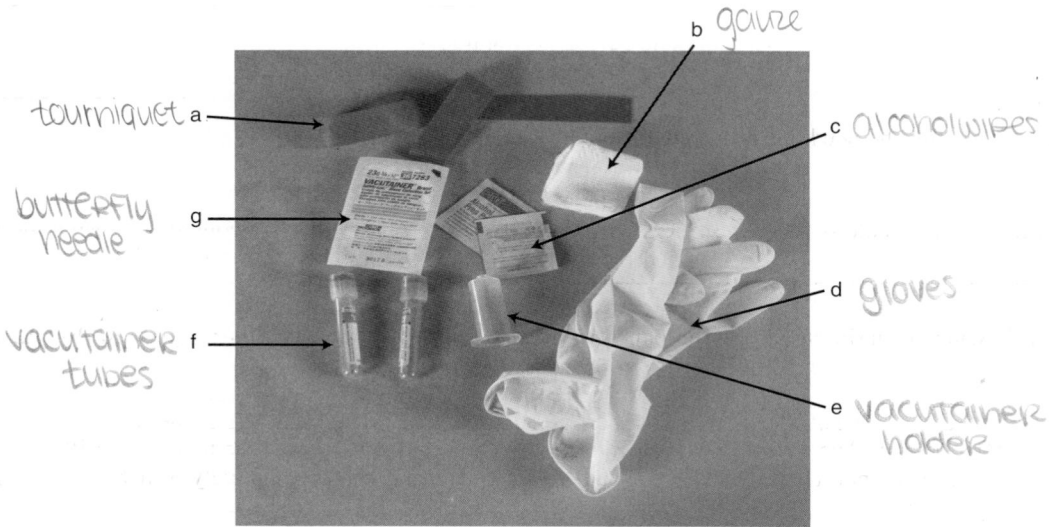

tourniquet a
b gauze
c alcohol wipes
butterfly needle g
vacutainer tubes f
d gloves
e vacutainer holder

69. Identify two quality assurance steps related to vacuum tube selection.

Check for any damages and check for expiration dates.

70. Discuss the Needle Stick Safety and Prevention Act passed by Congress, which directed the Occupational Safety and Health Administration (OSHA) to revise the bloodborne pathogens standards to require employers to identify and use safer medical devices.

It requires documenting the selection and evaluation of any new safety technology used by employees.

71. In the following case study steps, write **C** if the technique is correct or **I** if the technique is incorrect, and explain why in the space provided.
A medical assistant is performing a Vacutainer blood collection method.

I 1. The patient is told to sit on the end of the examination table.

Reclining position or sitting in a chair with arm support

I 2. The medical assistant washes his or her hands, puts on gloves, and then pops the top off of the index finger of the glove.

Do not pop the top of index finger of glove.

C 3. The tourniquet is applied, and the median cubital vein is determined for use; the tourniquet is then removed.

C 4. The chosen site is cleaned with 70% alcohol, working in concentric circles from the inside out, making sure to not backtrack. The tourniquet is then reapplied.

C 5. The nondominant hand anchors the vein.

I 6. The angle of the needle is 45 degrees as it enters the vein.

15 degrees

C 7. After the needle is removed, the safety device is immediately activated.

I 8. The needle is unscrewed from the holder and discarded in a sharps container, reusing the holder.

Discard everything in biohazard box.

72. In the following scenario about the venipuncture method, circle the incorrect techniques. In the space provided, explain the repercussions that could occur from using the incorrect method.

A medical assistant examines an arm to determine the correct vein to use to obtain blood. The arm has very small veins. The medical assistant decides to use the Vacutainer method. The patient's name is determined by asking, "Are you Mrs. Jones?" The patient is then told to sit in a chair with an arm. All the tubes that will be drawn on this patient are prelabeled before the draw. After putting on the tourniquet approximately 3 inches above the puncture site, the arm is cleaned with 70% isopropyl alcohol, starting at the puncture site and moving in a concentric circle outward. The site is retouched by the phlebotomist without cleaning the finger. The needle is inserted into the vein at a 15-degree angle. The lavender tube is filled first, followed by the red tube and gray tube; the green tube is filled last. After the last tube is filled, the needle is removed from the vein, and the tourniquet is removed. Tubes are mixed approximately three times and placed in an upright position in the tray to be quickly taken to the lab to perform analytical testing.

- asking, "Are you Mrs. Jones?" could be a different patient with same last name. - should be labeled after the blood is drawn. - order of draw is red, green, lavender, and gray. - tourniquet is removed before the needle is removed so the blood won't squirt out.

73. Label all the venipuncture supplies in the figure below (see Figure 4-22 in the textbook).

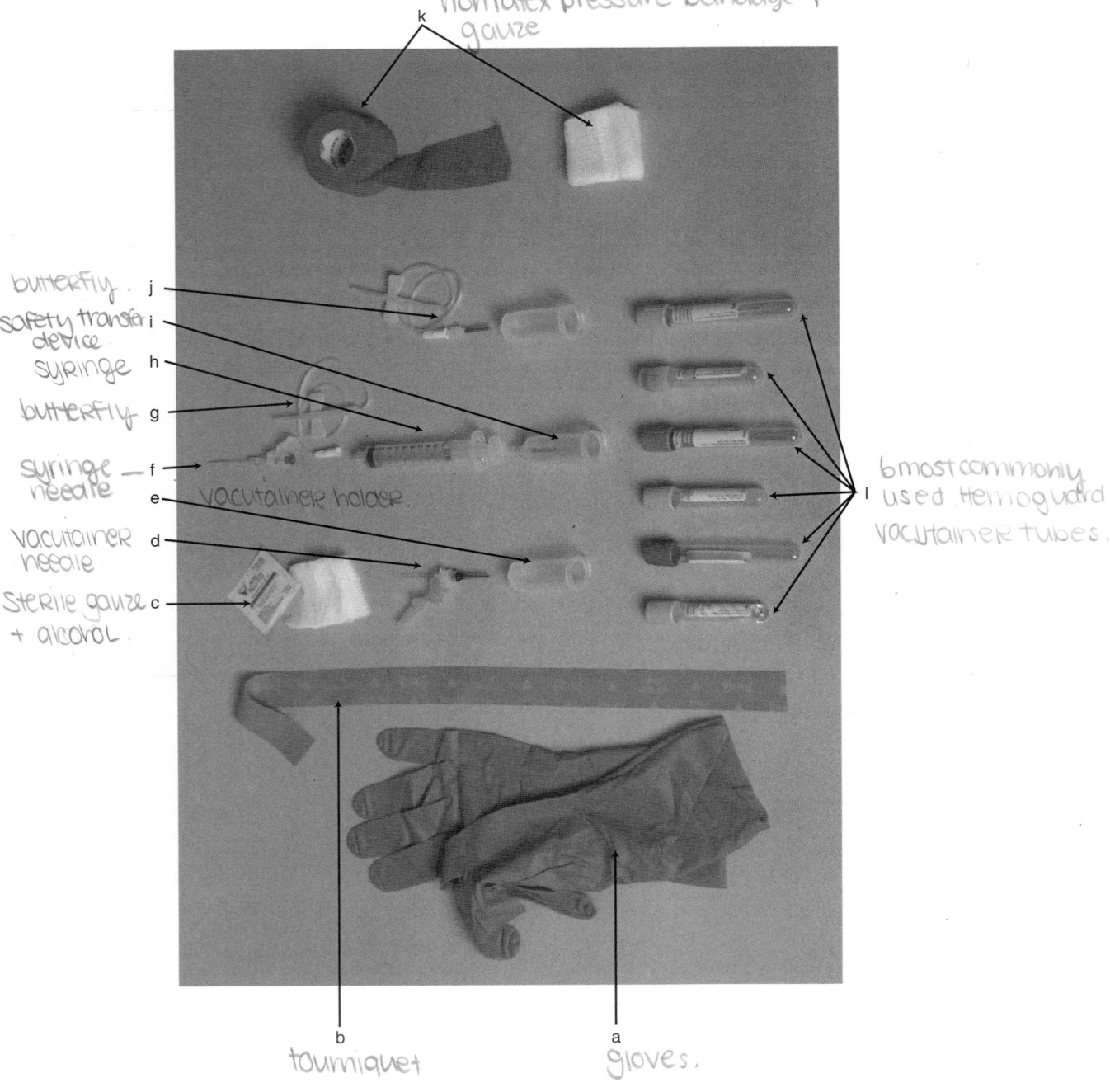

k — non latex pressure bandage + gauze

j — butterfly
i — safety transfer device
h — syringe
g — butterfly
f — syringe needle
e — vacutainer holder
d — vacutainer needle
c — sterile gauze + alcohol

l — 6 most commonly used Hemoguard vacutainer tubes.

b — tourniquet
a — gloves.

74. Internet activity: Visit one of the following Web sites, and present your findings to the class.

www.mchb.hrsa.gov (Maternal and Child Health Bureau of the Health Resources and Services Administration)

www.aap.org (American Academy of Pediatrics)

www.bd.com (Becton Dickinson)

www.nccls.org (National Committee for Clinical Laboratory Standards)

www.osha.gov (Occupational Safety and Health Administration)

75. The medical assistant is performing a Vacutainer procedure. The needle is inserted into the vein, and the vacuum tube is pushed into the Vacutainer holder. No blood is obtained. Discuss the possible reasons why this occurred.

The needle is not in a 15° angle, vein rolled, not where the vein
_is at._

76. During a venipuncture procedure, the patient becomes pale, sweats, and hyperventilates. Discuss what occurred and what should be done.

Syncope. Take the needle out, make the patient lie down, cold compress.

77. The plasma in the vacuum tube appears pink. Explain what this is, list three things that can cause it, and name three tests that can be affected by this condition.

Hemolysis. Vigorously shaking the tube, small needle, collapsing of vein.
Potassium, iron, and ammonia.

78. After a needle was inserted into a patient's vein, the patient experienced a tingling sensation radiating down the arm. What occurred, and what should the phlebotomist do?

needle hit a nerve. Move tourniquet and needle, apply pressure to the
site, and notify the physician.

Chapter **4** **Blood Collection**

Copyright © 2011, 2006 by Saunders, an imprint of Elsevier Inc. All rights reserved.

Procedure 4-1: Capillary Puncture Procedure

Person evaluated _____ Date _____

Evaluated by _____ Score _____

Outcome goal	To perform a capillary skin puncture with a retractable, nonreusable lancet
Conditions	Given the following supplies: - Sterile, disposable, retractable, nonreusable lancets (various lengths for the appropriate depth) - Microcollection containers, plastic capillary tubes (with anticoagulant) and sealers - Sterile gauze and 70% isopropyl alcohol pads in sterile packages - Gloves (latex and nonlatex for patients who are allergic) - Biohazard puncture-resistant sharps container - Warming devices, marking pen - Appropriate microcollection containers and/or testing devices depending on what test is ordered
Standards	Required time: 10 minutes Performance time _____ Total possible points = _____ Points earned = _____

Evaluation Rubric Codes:
S = Satisfactory, meets standard   **U** = Unsatisfactory, fails to meet standard

NOTE: Steps marked with an asterisk (*) are critical to achieve required competency.

Preparation	Scores	
	S	**U**
*1. Identified patient and placed in proper position.		
- Had patient state name.		
- Confirmed identification with patient (birth date or picture ID).		
- Compared with requisition.		
2. Sanitized hands and put on gloves.		
3. Determined the most suitable puncture site and warmed the site.		
- A finger stick: third and fourth finger should be used, making the puncture on the lateral part of the fingertip (slightly to the side of center) and perpendicular to the fingerprint.		
- Newborn or infant (not walking): the medial or lateral plantar section of the foot should be used.		
- Warmed area by massaging the areas five or six times or applied a warmed towel, preemie diaper, or a commercially available device to the site for 3 to 5 minutes.		

Procedure	Scores	
	S	**U**
*4. Disinfected area over chosen site and assembled equipment.		
- Cleaned the site with 70% alcohol.		
- Allowed to dry without fanning or blowing on cleansed site.		

	Scores	
	S	U
- Assembled the capillary equipment needed, determining the appropriate lancet device to use according to the age and amount of blood needed.		
- Placed all supplies in close proximity to hand.		
5. Pressing hard, made a puncture in the cleaned area at the appropriate site.		
*6. Wiped away the first drop of blood.		
*7. Collected the blood in the proper container by the correct technique.		
- Collected free-flowing drops of blood; did not scoop, scrape, or squeeze the site.		
- If blood was collected in a capillary tube, held the tube horizontal to the site and did not have any air bubbles.		
Follow-up	**Scores**	
	S	**U**
8. Asked the patient to apply pressure to site for 3 to 5 minutes.		
9. Gently mixed microcontainers by tilting 8 to 10 times and labeled all tubes properly.		
- Marked date and time of draw, patient name, and initials or name of phlebotomist.		
- Placed capillary tubes in a vacuum tube and labeled the vacuum tube.		
*10. Checked site for bleeding and applied pressure bandage to site.		
- If bleeding continued after 5 minutes, contacted physician.		
- Checked if patient was allergic to bandages before application.		
- Informed parent, if patient is a child, to remove the adhesive bandage after bleeding is stopped because children may choke on it if swallowed.		
11. Determined whether patient was feeling well before dismissing.		
*12. Completed proper documentation on patient chart (see below).		
*13. Properly performed disposal and disinfection.		
- Disposed all sharps into biohazard sharps containers.		
- Disposed regulated medical waste into biohazard bags (gloves, gauze).		
- Disinfected test area and instruments according to OSHA guidelines.		
14. Sanitized hands.		
Total Points per Column		

Patient Name: ＿＿＿＿＿＿＿＿＿

Patient Chart Entry: (Include when, what, how, why, any additional information, and the signature of the person charting.)

_____

_____

_____

Procedure 4-2: Heel Stick for Neonatal Screening Test Procedure

Person evaluated _____   Date _____

Evaluated by _____   Score _____

Outcome goal	Perform a capillary skin puncture with a retractable, nonreusable lancet
Conditions	Given the following supplies: - Gloves (preferably nonlatex for latex-sensitive patients) - Sterile gauze - Warming device - 70% isopropyl alcohol pads in sterile packages - Sterile, disposable, retractable, nonreusable neonatal lancets with no more than 2-mm depth - Neonatal screening filter paper
Standards	Required time: 15 minutes Performance time _____ Total possible points = _____ Points earned = _____

Evaluation Rubric Codes:
S = Satisfactory, meets standard   **U** = Unsatisfactory, fails to meet standard

NOTE: Steps marked with an asterisk (*) are critical to achieve required competency.

Preparation	Scores	
	S	**U**
*1. Wash the hands if they are visibly soiled. If not, use an alcohol-based rub for routine decontamination. Apply the hand rub to the palm of one hand, and rub the hands together, covering all surfaces until dry.		
2. Correctly identify the newborn by using the three-way match, and fill out all the information required on the card.		
3. Applied gloves.		
4. Choose the appropriate site for the heel stick according to the guidelines.		
- Newborn or infant (not walking): the medial or lateral plantar section of the foot should be used.		
- Applied a warmed towel, preemie diaper, or a commercially available device to the site for 3 to 5 minutes.		

Procedure	Scores	
	S	**U**
5. Clean the site with 70% isopropyl alcohol. Allow the alcohol to dry, and do not fan or blow on the site.		
6. With a gloved hand, place the lancet against the medial or lateral plantar surface of the heel of the foot.		
7. Place the blade slot area securely against the heel, and firmly and completely depress the lancet trigger.		
8. Gently wipe away the first drop of blood with sterile gauze or cotton ball.		
9. Apply gentle pressure with the thumb and ease intermittently as drops of blood form. Be sure to apply pressure in such a way that the incision site remains open.		

71

*10. The filter paper should be touched gently against the large blood drop, and in one step, a sufficient quantity of blood should soak through to completely fill a preprinted circle on the filter paper.		
- Do not reapply additional drops in the same circle.		
- The paper should not be pressed or smeared against the puncture site of the heel.		
- Blood should be applied only to one side of the filter paper, but both sides of the filter paper should be examined to ensure that the blood uniformly saturated the paper.		
11. After all five circles of blood have been collected from the heel of the newborn, the foot should be elevated above the body.		
NOTE: A minimum of three successful circles is needed by the laboratory to test for multiple metabolic disorders.		
12. A sterile gauze pad or cotton swab should be pressed against the puncture site until the bleeding stops.		
- It is not advisable to apply adhesive bandages over skin puncture sites on newborns.		

	Scores	
Follow-up	**S**	**U**
*13. Log and chart the procedure.		
14. Allow filter paper to dry thoroughly on a horizontal, level, nonabsorbent open surface for 3 hours at ambient temperature and away from direct sunlight.		
- Do not touch or smear blood on the filter paper, and do not contaminate the specimen card with cleaning chemicals or other substances.		
- Mail the thoroughly dried card (Fig. F in textbook) in the envelope provided by the health department.		
- Placed capillary tubes in a vacuum tube and labeled the vacuum tube.		
*15. Properly performed disposal and disinfection.		
- Disposed all sharps into biohazard sharps containers.		
- Disposed regulated medical waste into biohazard bags (gloves, gauze).		
- Disinfected test area and instruments according to OSHA guidelines.		
16. Sanitized hands.		
Total Points per Column		

Patient Name: _____

Patient Chart Entry: (Include when, what, how, why, any additional information, and the signature of the person charting.)

_____

_____

_____

Procedure 4-3: Vacutainer Method

Person evaluated _____   Date _____

Evaluated by _____   Score _____

Outcome goal	Perform a venipuncture by the Vacutainer method
Conditions	Given the following supplies: - Disposable gloves - Tourniquet - 70% isopropyl alcohol and sterile gauze pads - Vacutainer double-pointed needle and Vacutainer holder - Correct vacuum tubes for requested tests - Adhesive bandages - Test tube rack - Biohazard sharps containers and bags
Standards	Required time: 10 minutes Performance time _____ Total possible points = _____ Points earned = _____

Evaluation Rubric Codes:
S = Satisfactory, meets standard   **U** = Unsatisfactory, fails to meet standard

NOTE: Steps marked with an asterisk (*) are critical to achieve required competency.

Preparation	Scores S	Scores U
*1. Identified and placed patient in proper position.		
- Had patient state name.		
- Confirmed identification with patient (birth date or picture ID).		
- Compared identification with requisition.		
2. Sanitized hands and put on gloves.		
3. Applied tourniquet and determined the most suitable puncture site.		
- Used sufficient pressure to stop venous flow but not arterial flow.		
- Palpated and determined size, depth, and direction of vein.		
4. Removed tourniquet, disinfected area over chosen site, and assembled equipment.		
- Cleansed the site with 70% alcohol in concentric circles from inside out.		
- Allowed to dry without fanning or blowing on cleansed site.		
- Connected the venipuncture assembly in a sterile manner.		
- Placed all supplies in close proximity to arm.		

Procedure	Scores	
	S	U
5. Reapplied tourniquet and instructed patient to make a fist (no pumping).		
*6. Disinfected gloved fingers if necessary to palpate site again.		
*7. Uncovered needle, anchored vein, and inserted needle.		
- Pulled skin taut with nondominant thumb 1 to 2 inches below and to the side of the puncture site.		
- Inserted needle ¼ to ½ inches distal to the vein with bevel up in one swift, continuous motion with dominant hand.		
*8. Pushed tube into needle holder.		
- Used the index and middle fingers of nondominant hand on both sides of the flange and pushed the tube with the thumb of the same hand.		
*9. Followed proper order of draw when filling, removing, and mixing the tubes.		
- Used thumb of nondominant hand against flange and pulled tube out with the fingers of the same hand.		
- Inverted each tube gently to mix blood with additives.		
- Removed the last tube to prevent blood dripping from needle.		
- Instructed patient to release fist.		
*10. Removed tourniquet before taking needle out of arm.		
*11. Placed sterile gauze over needle as it was pulled out and then applied pressure to site.		
- Did not press on the gauze until *after* the needle was removed.		
*12. Immediately activated needle safety device and discarded Vacutainer and needle as a unit into the sharps container.		

Follow-up	Scores	
	S	U
13. Asked the patient to apply pressure to site for 3 to 5 minutes.		
14. Gently mixed tubes by tilting 8 to 10 times and labeled all tubes properly.		
- Marked patient name, date and time of draw, and initials or name of phlebotomist.		
*15. Checked site for bleeding and applied pressure bandage to site.		
- If bleeding continued after 5 minutes, contacted physician.		
- Checked if patient was allergic to bandages before application.		
16. Determined if patient was feeling well before dismissing.		
17. Completed proper documentation on patient chart (see following page).		

*18. Properly disposed and disinfected materials.		
- Disposed all sharps into biohazard sharp containers.		
- Disposed regulated medical waste (e.g., gloves, gauze) into biohazard bags.		
- Disinfected test area and instruments according to OSHA guidelines.		
19. Sanitized hands.		
Total Points per Column		

Patient Name: _____

Patient Chart Entry: (Include when, what, how, why, any additional information, and the signature of the person charting.)

_____

_____

_____

Procedure 4-4: Syringe Method

Person evaluated _____   Date _____

Evaluated by _____   Score_____

Outcome goal	Perform a venipuncture by the syringe method
Conditions	Given the following supplies: - Disposable gloves - Tourniquet - 70% isopropyl alcohol and sterile gauze pads - Proper-sized syringe and needle - Safety transfer device - Correct vacuum tubes for requested tests - Adhesive bandages - Test tube rack - Biohazard sharps containers and bags
Standards	Required time: 10 minutes Performance time _____ Total possible points = _____ Points earned = _____

Evaluation Rubric Codes:
S = Satisfactory, meets standard   **U** = Unsatisfactory, fails to meet standard

NOTE: Steps marked with an asterisk (*) are critical to achieve required competency.

Preparation	Scores	
	S	**U**
*1. Identified and placed patient in proper position.		
- Had patient state name.		
- Confirmed identification with patient (birth date or picture ID).		
- Compared identification with requisition.		
2. Sanitized hands and put on gloves.		
3. Applied tourniquet and determined the most suitable puncture site.		
- Applied sufficient pressure to stop venous flow but not arterial flow.		
- Palpated and determined size, depth, and direction of vein.		
4. Removed tourniquet, disinfected area over chosen site, and assembled equipment.		
- Cleaned the site with 70% alcohol in concentric circles from inside out.		
- Allowed to dry without fanning or blowing on cleansed site.		
- Connected the syringe assembly in a sterile manner.		
- Placed all supplies in close proximity to arm.		

Procedure	Scores	
	S	**U**
*5. Reapplied tourniquet and instructed patient to make a fist (no pumping).		
- Disinfected gloved fingers if necessary to palpate site again.		

	S	U
*6. Removed needle cover, anchored vein, and inserted needle.		
- Pulled skin taut with nondominant thumb 1 to 2 inches distal to the site of the puncture.		
- Inserted needle ¼ to ½ inches distal to the vein with bevel up in one swift, continuous motion with dominant hand at the appropriate angle.		
*7. Gently pulled syringe plunger back.		
- Was careful to not pull out of the vein.		
- Instructed patient to release fist.		
*8. Removed tourniquet before taking needle out of arm.		
*9. Placed sterile gauze over needle as it was pulled out, then applied pressure to site.		
- Did not press on the gauze until after the needle was removed.		
*10. Immediately activated syringe needle safety device, unscrewed the needle, and discarded it into the sharps container.		

Follow-up	Scores	
	S	U
11. Asked the patient to apply pressure with gauze to site for 3 to 5 minutes.		
12. Filled the vacuum tubes in the proper order of draw by using a transfer safety device.		
- Did not push on the plunger.		
13. Gently mixed tubes by tilting 8 to 10 times and labeled all tubes properly.		
- Marked patient name, date and time of draw, and initials or name of phlebotomist.		
*14. Checked site for bleeding and applied pressure bandage to site.		
- If bleeding continued after 5 minutes, contacted physician.		
- Checked if patient was allergic to bandages before application.		
15. Determined if patient was feeling well before dismissing.		
16. Completed proper documentation on patient chart (see below).		
*17. Properly disposed and disinfected materials.		
- Disposed all sharps, including the transfer device/syringe, into biohazard sharps container.		
- Disposed regulated medical waste into biohazard bags (gloves, gauze).		
- Disinfected test area and instruments according to OSHA guidelines.		
18. Sanitized hands.		
Total Points per Column		

Patient Name _____

Patient Chart Entry: (Include when, what, how, why, any additional information, and the signature of the person charting.)

_____

_____

_____

Procedure 4-5: Two Butterfly Methods from a Hand and Training Model

Person evaluated _____ Date _____

Evaluated by _____ Score _____

Outcome goal	Perform a venipuncture by the butterfly method
Conditions	Given the following supplies: - Disposable gloves, tourniquet, 70% isopropyl alcohol and gauze pads - Winged butterfly set (Safety-Lock and/or Push Button) with syringe adapter and Vacutainer adapter - Proper-sized syringe or Vacutainer holder - Correct vacuum tubes for requested tests - Adhesive bandages - Test tube rack and biohazard sharps containers and bags
Standards	Required time: 10 minutes Performance time _____ Total possible points = _____ Points earned = _____
Evaluation Rubric Codes: **S** = Satisfactory, meets standard **U** = Unsatisfactory, fails to meet standard	
NOTE: Steps marked with an asterisk (*) are critical to achieve required competency.	

Preparation	Scores	
	S	**U**
*1. Identified and placed patient in proper position.		
- Had patient state name.		
- Confirmed identification with patient (birth date or picture ID).		
- Compared identification with requisition.		
2. Sanitized hands and put on gloves.		
3. Applied tourniquet and determined the most suitable puncture site.		
- Applied sufficient pressure to stop venous flow but not arterial flow.		
- Palpated and determined size, depth, and direction of vein.		
4. Removed tourniquet, disinfected area over chosen site, and assembled equipment.		
- Cleaned the site with 70% alcohol in concentric circles from inside out.		
- Allowed to dry without fanning or blowing on cleansed site.		
- Straightened out the butterfly tubing.		
- Connected the venipuncture butterfly assembly in a sterile manner to a syringe or a Vacutainer holder.		
- Pushed the plunger back and forth to break the seal if attaching a syringe.		
- Placed all supplies in close proximity to arm or hand.		

Chapter **4** **Blood Collection**

Procedure	Scores	
	S	U
*5. Reapplied the tourniquet and disinfected gloved fingers if necessary to palpate site again.		
*6. Removed needle sheath, anchored vein, and inserted needle.		
- Pulled skin taut with nondominant thumb 1 to 2 inches below and to the side of the puncture site.		
- Held the butterfly wings together with the dominant hand and inserted needle ¼ to ½ inches distal to the vein with bevel up in one swift, continuous motion with dominant hand at the appropriate angle.		
*7. Used the correct technique to obtain blood.		
- Gently pulled syringe plunger back if using syringe method.		
- Used the index and middle fingers of nondominant hand on both sides of the flange and pushed the tube into the holder with the thumb of the same hand if the Vacutainer method was used.		
*8. Tourniquet removed before taking needle out of arm.		
*9. Placed sterile gauze over needle as it was pulled out and then applied pressure to the site.		
- Did not press on the gauze until after the needle was removed.		
*10. Immediately activated butterfly needle safety device in a safe manner and disposed of butterfly apparatus properly (illustrations show how to activate the Safety Lock and the Push Button safety devices).		
- If Vacutainer method was used, the butterfly needle, tubing, and Vacutainer holder were placed in a biohazard sharps container.		
- If a syringe method was used, the syringe was removed from the butterfly tubing, and the butterfly needle and tubing were discarded into a biohazard sharps container.		

Follow-up	Scores	
	S	U
11. Asked the patient to apply pressure with gauze to site for 3 to 5 minutes.		
12. Filled the vacuum tubes in the proper order of draw by using a transfer safety device if syringe method was used.		
- Did not push on plunger; let vacuum fill the tube.		
13. Gently mixed tubes by tilting 8 to 10 times, and labeled all tubes properly.		
- Marked patient name, date and time of draw, and initials or name of phlebotomist.		
*14. Checked site for bleeding and applied pressure bandage to site.		
- If bleeding continued after 5 minutes, contacted physician.		
- Checked if patient was allergic to bandages before application.		
15. Determined if patient was feeling well before dismissing.		
16. Completed proper documentation on patient chart (see following page).		

*17. Properly disposed and disinfected equipment.		
- Disposed all sharps, including the transfer device and syringe (if syringe method was used), into biohazard sharps containers.		
- Disposed regulated medical waste (e.g., gloves, gauze) into biohazard bags.		
- Disinfected test area and instruments according to OSHA guidelines.		
18. Sanitized hands.		
Total Points per Column		

Patient Name: _____

Patient Chart Entry: (Include when, what, how, why, any additional information, and the signature of the person charting.)

_____

_____

_____

Vacuum Tube Exercise

Visualize the following picture:
- *Blue* sky is at the top and is the first tube to draw.
- The *red and gold* rays of the sun are on the horizon. They both must be drawn *after* the blue but *before* the remaining anticoagulant tubes.
- *Green* grassy hill is located below the sun rays.
- *Lavender* flowers are at the bottom of the hill growing above the rocks.
- *Gray* rocks are at the bottom of the picture because gray is the last tube to draw.

   Next, fill in the blank boxes and missing words from Table 4-5 in the textbook. Cut the rows, mix them up, and then place back in order, or cut all the boxes and put them back together like a puzzle.

Colors of Picture and the Plastic Vacutainer Tubes Placed in Order of Draw from Top to Bottom		Additives	Laboratory Uses
blue _____	blue topped	_____	_____
red rays and gold _____	topped _____ _____	clot activator in plastic tubes (red *glass* tubes do not have clot activator)	both yield serum commonly used for testing blood _____
	gold topped _____	_____ and _____	
_____ grass	green topped	_____ (with lithium or sodium)	special tests such as _____
lavender flowers	lavender topped	_____	_____
gray _____	_____	oxalate	for _____ testing

5 Hematology

VOCABULARY REVIEW

Match each hematology term with the correct definition.

A. anisocytosis
B. baso
C. differentiate
D. eosin
E. erythroblasts
F. formed elements
G. granulocytes

H. hematologists
I. hematopoiesis
J. hemocytoblast
K. macrophages
L. megakaryocyte
M. myeloblast

N. nongranulocytes
O. -phil
P. poikilocytosis
Q. polymorphonuclear
R. reticulocytes
S. thrombocytes

____l.____ 1. Large nuclear cell in the bone marrow that fragments its cytoplasm to become platelets

____m.____ 2. Stem cell that develops into the three kinds of granulocytes

____p.____ 3. Abnormally shaped

____d.____ 4. Acid

____b____ 5. Alkaline

____e.____ 6. Also called rubriblasts, which become red blood cells

____o.____ 7. Attraction

____i.____ 8. Blood production

____f.____ 9. Cells and cell fragments that can be viewed under the microscope

____h.____ 10. Specialists who evaluate the cellular elements of blood microscopically and analytically

____k.____ 11. Large, engulfing cells in the tissues that come from monocytes

____n.____ 12. Lymphocyte and monocyte group

____q.____ 13. Many-shaped nucleus; also called PMN or seg

____g.____ 14. Neutrophils, basophils, and eosinophils group

____r.____ 15. Newly released red blood cells in the blood that still contain some nuclear DNA

____j.____ 16. Stem cell capable of becoming any of the blood cells

____c.____ 17. To change and become something different

____a.____ 18. Variances in red blood cell size

____s.____ 19. Platelets

Match each coagulation or pathology term with the correct definition.

A. anemia	G. leukemia	M. rouleaux formation
B. embolus	H. leukocytosis	N. thrombosis
C. fibrinogen, prothrombin	I. leukopenia	O. vitamin K
D. hemolysis	J. polycythemia	P. differential count
E. hemostasis	K. red blood cell indices	Q. polychromia
F. hypoxemia	L. coagulation	

___O.___ 20. A critical element in the production of prothrombin

___b.___ 21. A traveling clot

___J.___ 22. Abnormal condition of increased red blood cells

___I.___ 23. Abnormal decrease in white blood cells

___h.___ 24. Abnormal increase in white blood cells

___N.___ 25. Abnormal condition of clotting

___a.___ 26. Condition in which the red blood cell or hemoglobin levels are below normal

___d.___ 27. Destruction of the red blood cells

___f.___ 28. Lack of oxygen in the blood

___m.___ 29. Like stacked chips

___k.___ 30. Mathematic ratios of the three red blood cell tests (hemoglobin, hematocrit, and red blood cell count)

___e.___ 31. Blood's ability to maintain the balance of initiating a clotting response to stop bleeding and at the same time prevent the blood from forming an unwanted stationary clot

___C.___ 32. Two plasma proteins involved in clotting

___P.___ 33. Percentage of the five kinds of white blood cells

___g.___ 34. Cancer of the white blood cells

___q.___ 35. Increase in color (based on hemoglobin concentration)

___l.___ 36. Process of clotting

FUNDAMENTAL CONCEPTS

37. Blood collected from a ___vein___ or a ___capillary___ may be used for routine hematologic procedures.

38. The anticoagulated Vacutainer tube containing ___EDTA___ with a ___lavender___ top is used for most hematology tests.

39. Match each blood component with its associated characteristic.

___d.___ basophil

___f.___ erythrocyte

___g.___ monocyte

___a.___ neutrophil

___e.___ platelet

___C.___ lymphocyte

___b.___ eosinophil

A. Able to engulf foreign matter, especially bacteria
B. Increases in number during allergic reactions
C. Can differentiate into a T cell or B cell
D. Enters the tissues to mediate the inflammatory response
E. Gathers around the site of a damaged blood vessel and releases chemicals to stimulate clot formation
F. Carries oxygen from the lungs to the cells of the body
G. Becomes a macrophage when it leaves the blood to clean up debris in the tissues

Chapter 5 Hematology

Copyright © 2011, 2006 by Saunders, an imprint of Elsevier Inc. All rights reserved.

40. Label the missing elements of the following hematopoiesis chart (see Figure 5-3 in the textbook). pg 131

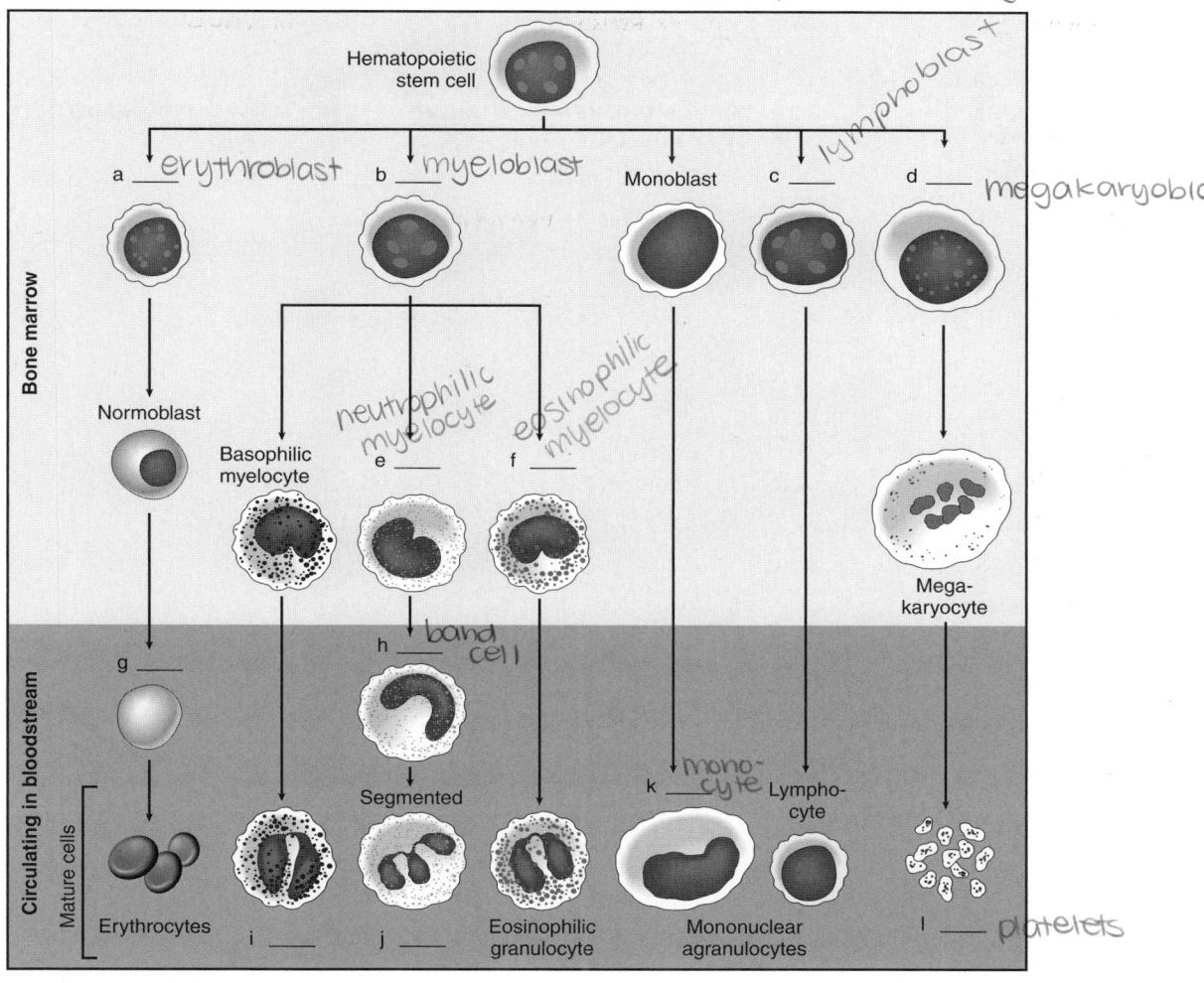

Preparation of a Blood Smear

41. A properly done blood smear will have a _____feathered_____ edge at the thin end of the slide and a section containing well-distributed blood cells in the _____body_____ of the slide.

42. Blood smears are observed under the _____oil immersion_____ lens.

43. When identifying cells, what three characteristics should the technician observe? (Hint: *The RBC Atlas* and *WBC Atlas* describe the general characteristics to observe in blood cells.)

_____Size, shape, color_____

_____

Hemostasis

44. Explain the involvement of each of the following as they pertain to hemostasis.

Blood vessels _____constricts, slowing down the blood flow_____

Platelets _____concentrates around the damaged site and initiate a clot made of fibrin mesh._____

Clotting factors _____(13) begin a chain reaction to form fibrin initiate a clot_____

Anticoagulants _____(heparin) to keep clotting mechanism in balance_____

Chapter **5** **Hematology**

45. What is the difference between a thrombus and an embolus? __Thrombus is a unwanted station-__
__ary clot and embolus is a releasing a traveling clot.__

PROCEDURES: CLINICAL LABORATORY IMPROVEMENT AMENDMENT (CLIA)–WAIVED HEMATOLOGY TESTS

Hemoglobin

46. The two main components of hemoglobin are ___heme (iron)___ and ___globin (protein)___.

47. What is the function of hemoglobin? ___to bind the oxygen in the RBCs.___

Hematocrit

48. Match the following average hematocrit percentages to each population, and note the highest to the lowest averages.

   __b.__ Normal average hematocrit for women   a. 56%

   __c__ Normal average hematocrit for a 6-year-old child   b. 42%

   __d.__ Normal average hematocrit for men   c. 38%

   __a.__ Normal average hematocrit for newborns   d. 47%

49. If a sample of capillary blood is used for the microhematocrit, the capillary tube must contain a(n)
___anticoagulant___.

50. One condition in which a low hematocrit value may be found is ___anemia___.

51. True or false: Spun hematocrits should be performed in duplicate. ___true___

52. Label the layers of the spun hematocrit tube.

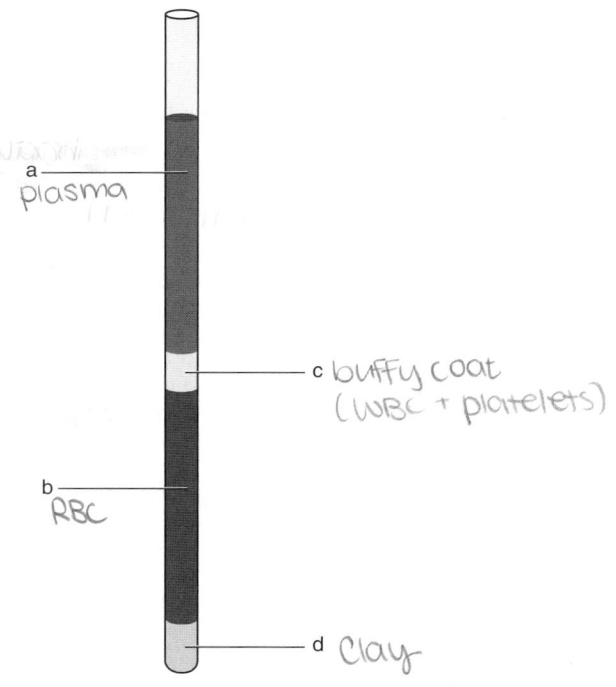

a — plasma

c buffy coat (WBC + platelets)

b — RBC

d clay

Erythrocyte Sedimentation Rate

53. What medical conditions can cause an increased erythrocyte sedimentation rate?
    Inflammatory diseases, autoimmune diseases, carcinomas,
    and certain forms of leukemia.

54. What technical interferences would cause an increased erythrocyte sedimentation rate?
    False increased rates, false decreased rates, vibrating surface,

Prothrombin Time

55. Describe the role of prothrombin in blood coagulation.
    It screens for patient who lack clotting factors, liver disease, or deficient
    in vitamin k. Its prone to bleeding in patient with PT.

56. Explain the major use of the prothrombin time test. _PT test uses thromboplastin as the_
    active reagent to initiate the coagulation process.
    *anticoagulant therapy in patients

57. Match each test with its reference range.
    _C._ hemoglobin   a. 36% to 55%
    _a._ hematocrit   b. 0 to 20 mm/hr
    _d._ ProTime   c. 12 to 18 g/dL
    _b._ ESR   d. approx. 9 to 18 seconds, or 2 to 2.5 INR

58. Label the Hemocue equipment and supplies (see Procedure 5-2 in the textbook).

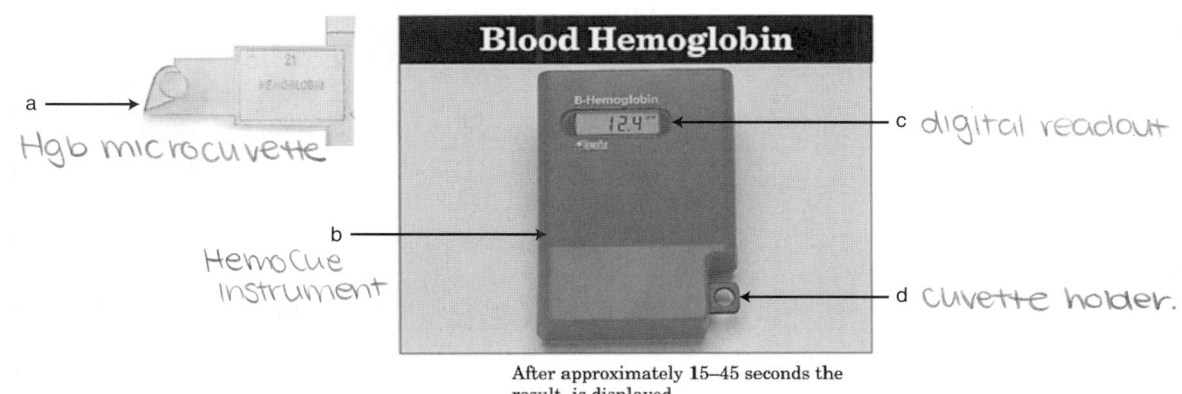

a → Hgb microcuvette

b → HemoCue Instrument

c digital readout

d cuvette holder.

Blood Hemoglobin

After approximately 15–45 seconds the result is displayed.

59. Label the SEDIPLAST ESR supplies (see Procedure 5-5 in the textbook).

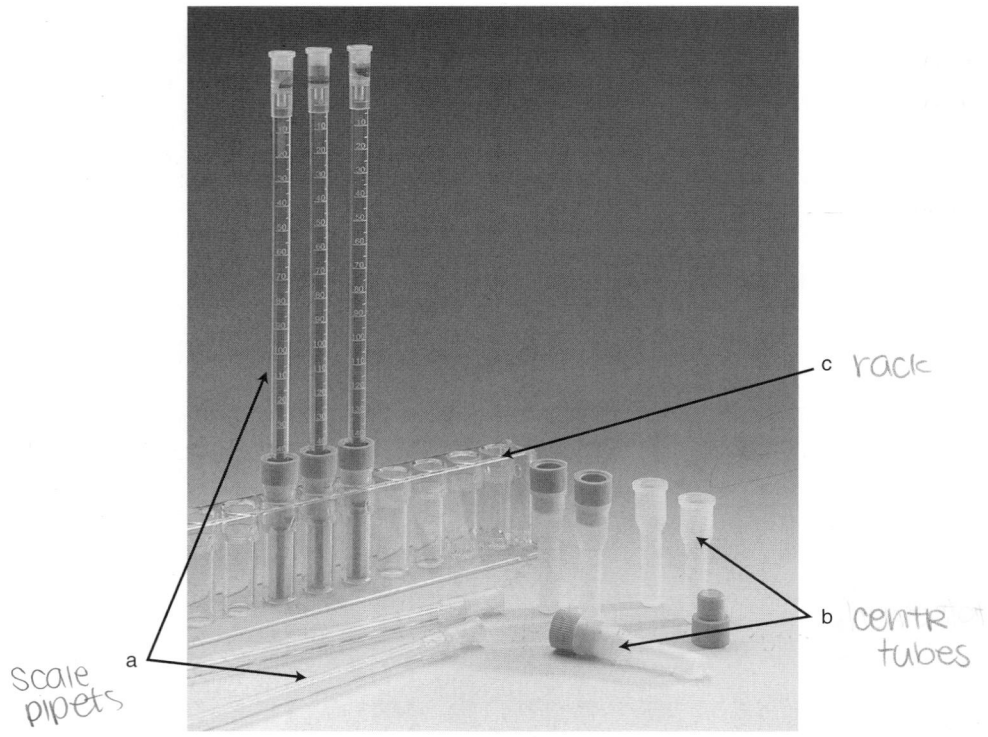

c rack

b centR tubes

a scale pipets

ADVANCED CONCEPTS: COMPLETE BLOOD COUNT

60. List the seven tests involved in the complete blood count.

Red blood cell count

Hematocrit

Hemoglobin

RBC indexes

WBCs count

Differential WC count

Platelet count.

61. What changes in blood cell size are caused by deficiency of vitamin B_{12}? (Hint: Look under "Anemias" in the textbook.)

Pernicious anemia. Cells appears enlarged, fragile, and abnormally shaped.

62. List two conditions in which anisocytosis is found. (Hint; Look under "Anemias" in the textbook.)

Aplastic anemia, pernicious anemia

63. Match the red blood cell indexes to their reference ranges. (Hint: See Table 5-3 or 5-4, and note the units associated with each test.)

   c. MCV   a. 26 to 34 pg

   a. MCH   b. 31% to 37% or g/dL

   b. MCHC   c. 82 to 98 μm^3 or fL

64. Hypochromic, microcytic red blood cells have a (higher or lower) ____lower____ MCV and (higher or lower) ____lower____ MCHC.

65. Why does anemia or thrombocytopenia develop in patients with leukemia? (Hint: Consider where and how hematopoiesis occurs.)

____Leukemia patients have more RBCs then WBC because the bone____
____marrow sends out cells before it____

66. Name one cause of eosinophilia. (Review granulocyte functions in "Fundamental Concepts.")

____Allergic Reaction.____

67. Name one cause of neutrophilia. (Review granulocyte functions in "Fundamental Concepts.")

____ability to engulf and digest foreign matter, especially____
____, pathogenic bacteria.____

70. Match the cell with its differential reference percentage according to Table 5-3 in your textbook, and note the highest to the lowest.

   c. band   a. 3% to 9%

   e. lymphocyte   b. 50% to 65%

   b. neutrophil   c. 0% to 7%

   a. monocyte   d. 0% to 1%

   f. eosinophil   e. 25% to 40%

   d. basophil   f. 1% to 3%

92

Chapter **5** Hematology

Procedure 5-1: Diff Staining Procedure

Person evaluated _____ Date _____

Evaluated by _____ Score _____

Outcome goal	Demonstrate the proper staining of a blood smear
Conditions	Given the following supplies: - Quick Diff stain: fixative, red eosin dye, blue baso dye; - staining rack; - water source (bottled or running water); - bibulous paper - Personal protective equipment – gown & gloves
Standards	Required time: 10 minutes Performance time _____ Total possible points = _____ Points earned = _____
Evaluation Rubric Codes: **S** = Satisfactory, meets standard **U** = Unsatisfactory, fails to meet standard	

Preparation	Scores	
	S	**U**
1. Put on personal protective equipment (PPE).		

Procedure	Scores	
	S	**U**
2. Dip the slide in fixative three to five times and allow it to dry completely.		
3. Dip the slide into the red eosin dye three to five times.		
4. Let the excess dye run off and blot the rest away with absorbent paper.		
5. Dip the slide into the blue baso dye three to five times.		
6. After the blue dye is blotted away, rinse the slide thoroughly with water on both sides and allow it to air dry. It may also be pressed between two bibulous papers to help remove the water.		

Follow-up	Scores	
	S	**U**
*7. Observe the slide under the oil immersion lens of the microscope. The challenge is to find the WBCs.		
- Refer to the microscope skill sheet 2-1 in Chapter 2 for the proper steps to bring the slide into focus under the oil immersion lens.		
- The cells and platelets will be enlarged 1000 times (100× oil objective times the 10× ocular lens).		
- The slide will show predominantly RBCs with some small platelet clumps throughout.		
- The two most commonly found WBCs are segmented neutrophils and small lymphocytes.		
- See Table 5-1 for assistance in identifying the WBCs.		
Total Points per Column		

Procedure 5-4: Hematocrit: HemataSTAT Method

Person evaluated _____ Date _____

Evaluated by _____ Score _____

Outcome goal	To perform FDA-approved hematocrit waived test following the most current OSHA safety guidelines and applying the correct quality control
Conditions	Supplies required: - Plastic capillary pipettes with anticoagulant - Sealant clay (i.e., Critoseal) - Liquid controls: high and low - Gloves, gown, alcohol, gauze, and lancets
Standards	Required time = 15 minutes Performance time = _____ Total possible points = _____ Points earned = _____
Evaluation Rubric Codes: **S** = Satisfactory, meets standard **U** = Unsatisfactory, fails to meet standard	
NOTE: Steps marked with an asterisk (*) are critical to achieve required competency.	

Preparation: Preanalytical Phase	Scores	
	S	**U**
A. Test information		
- Kit or instrument method: **HemataSTAT II**		
- Manufacturer: **Separation Technology, Inc. (STI)**		
- Proper storage (e.g., temperature, light): **room temperature**		
- Expiration date: (**2 years or 30 days after opened**)		
- Package insert or test flow chart available: _____ yes _____ no		
B. Specimen information		
- Type of specimen: **capillary blood or venous blood in EDTA tube**		
- Specimen testing device: **two capillary tubes filled at least halfway**		
C. Personal protective equipment: **gloves, gown, face shield**		
D. Assembled all the above, sanitized hands, and applied personal protective equipment.		
Procedure: Analytical Phase	Scores	
	S	**U**
E. Performed/observed quality control		
1. Quantitative testing controls		
- **HemataCHEK reference control**		
- Control levels: high _____ low _____ normal _____		

	S	U
F. Perform patient test		
1. Followed proper steps (from test flow chart).		
2. Collected whole blood into capillary tubes and sealed one end by pressing and turning in sealant, and then tapped the sealed end. Or, held self-sealant tube vertical for 15 seconds.		
3. Inserted the sealed end of capillary tube into the HemataSTAT rotor tube holder.		
4. Closed centrifuge lid, locked latch, and pressed "RUN" to spin for 60 seconds.		
5. Waited for beeps, then unlocked latch and opened lid.		
6. Moved slider and sealed end of capillary tube to far left side of reader tray and rotated tube so entire "RED CELL/PLASMA" diagonal interface could be seen.		
7. Pressed "ENT" to read tube.		
8. Moved the slider black line to "SEALANT/RED CELL" interface and pressed "ENT."		
9. Moved the slider black line to "RED CELL/PLASMA" interface and pressed "ENT."		
10. Moved slider black line to "PLASMA/AIR" interface, pressed "ENT," noted result.		
11. Repeated steps 6 to 10 with second tube.		
- Result must be within 2% agreement of first reading.		
- Recorded the average of the two readings.		

*Accurate Results _____   Instructor Confirmation _____

Follow-up: Postanalytical Phase	Scores	
	S	U
*G. Proper documentation		
1. On control log: _____ yes _____ no		
2. On patient log: _____ yes _____ no		
3. Documented on patient chart (see following page).		
4. Identified critical values and took appropriate steps to notify physician.		
- Hematocrit expected values: Adult men = 42% to 52% Adult women = 36% to 48% Infants = 32% to 38% Children = increase to adult levels		
H. Proper disposal and disinfection		
1. Disposed all sharps into biohazard sharps containers.		
2. Disposed all other regulated medical waste into biohazard bags.		
3. Disinfected test area and instruments according to OSHA guidelines.		
4. Sanitized hands after removing gloves.		
Totals Counts per Column		

Patient Name: _____

Patient Chart Entry: (Include when, what, why, any additional information, and the signature of the person charting.)

_____

_____

Procedure 5-5: ESR: SEDIPLAST System Procedure

Person evaluated _____ Date _____

Evaluated by _____ Score _____

Outcome goal	To perform FDA-approved ESR waived test following the most current OSHA safety guidelines and applying the correct quality control
Conditions	Supplies needed: - Plastic Westergren pipette graduated from 0 to 200 mm - SEDIPLAST vials with citrate diluent - Westergren rack for holding the pipettes - Disposal transfer pipette - Timer - Gloves, gown, face shield
Standards	Required time = 70 minutes Performance time = _____ Total possible points = _____ Points earned = _____

Evaluation Rubric Codes:
S = Satisfactory, meets standard   **U** = Unsatisfactory, fails to meet standard

NOTE: Steps marked with an asterisk (*) are critical to achieve required competency.

Preparation: Preanalytical Phase	Scores	
	S	U
A. Test information		
- Kit or instrument method: **SEDIPLAST**		
- Manufacturer: **Polymedco, Inc.**		
- Proper storage (e.g., temperature, light): **room temperature**		
- Lot number on package: _____		
- Expiration date: _____		
- Package insert or test flow chart available: _____ yes _____ no		
B. Personal protective equipment: **gloves, gown, face shield**		
C. Proper specimen used for test		
- Type of specimen: **fresh EDTA whole blood up to 2 hours or refrigerated blood up to 6 hours**		
- Specimen testing device: **SEDIPLAST vial and pipette**		
D. Assembled all the above, sanitized hands, and applied personal protective equipment.		
Procedure: Analytical Phase	Scores	
	S	U
E. Performed/observed quality control methods: not applicable.		
F. Performed patient test.		

1. Removed stopper on vial and filled the vial with blood to indicated mark with a disposable transfer pipette (0.8 mL of blood needed).		
2. Replaced vial stopper and inverted vial several times to mix.		
3. Placed vial in SEDIPLAST rack on a level surface free of vibrations and jarring.		
4. Pressed the disposable SEDIPLAST pipette gently through the stopper with a twisting motion and continued to press until the pipette rested on the bottom of the vial (the pipette auto-zeros the blood, and any excess flows into the closed reservoir compartment at the top of the pipette).		
5. Set the timer for 1 hour, and let specimen stand undisturbed.		
6. After 1 hour read the numeric results of the ESR (used the scale at the top of the pipette to measure the distance from the top of the plasma to the top of the red blood cells).		

*Accurate Results _____   Instructor Confirmation _____

Follow-up: Postanalytical Phase	Scores	
	S	U
*G. Proper documentation		
1. On patient log: _____ yes _____ no		
2. Documented on patient chart (see below).		
3. Identified critical values, and took appropriate steps to notify physician.		
- ESR expected values: Men < 50 years = 0 to 15 mm/hr Men > 50 years = 0 to 20 mm/hr Women < 50 years = 0 to 20 mm/hr Women > 50 years = 0 to 30 mm/hr		
H. Proper disposal and disinfection		
1. Disposed all sharps into biohazard sharps containers.		
2. Disposed all other regulated medical waste into biohazard bags.		
3. Disinfected test area and instruments according to OSHA guidelines.		
4. Sanitized hands after removing gloves.		
Totals Counts per Column		

Patient name: _____

Patient Chart Entry: (Include when, what, why, any additional information, and the signature of the person charting.)

_____

_____

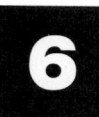 **Chemistry**

VOCABULARY REVIEW

Match each definition with the correct term.

___t.___ 1. endogenous cholesterol

___s.___ 2. glycogen

___h___ 3. exogenous cholesterol

___a.___ 4. catalysts

___m___ 5. hyperinsulinemia

___c.___ 6. glycosylated Hgb

___p.___ 7. hyperlipidemia

___N___ 8. insulin

___R___ 9. glucagon

___i___ 10. trans fats

___l.___ 11. ions

___g.___ 12. glycosuria

___e.___ 13. atherosclerosis

___b___ 14. panels

___d.___ 15. dyslipidemia

___F.___ 16. carbohydrates

___u.___ 17. definitive diagnosis

___J___ 18. hyperglycemia

___O___ 19. clinical diagnosis

___q___ 20. ketoacidosis

___K___ 21. noncarbohydrate energy sources

A. Chemicals that produce specific changes in other substances without being changed themselves

B. Groups of tests providing information on particular organs or body metabolism

C. Glucose permanently changes the hemoglobin molecule within red blood cells

D. Abnormal fat levels in the blood

E. Formation of plaque along the inside walls of blood vessels

F. Sugars and starches

G. Sugar in the urine

H. Cholesterol derived from the diet

I. Man-made hydrogenated fats

J. Elevated blood sugar

K. Fats and proteins that are able to convert to glucose if necessary

L. Electrolytes consisting of positively or negatively charged particles

M. Excessively high blood insulin levels

N. Hormone produced by the pancreas to lower blood glucose

O. Diagnosis based on the patient's initial signs and symptoms

P. Excessive fat in blood, giving a milky appearance in the plasma

Q. Condition of excessive ketones in the blood causing an acid condition

R. Hormone produced by the pancreas to raise blood glucose

S. Stored form of glucose especially found in muscles and the liver

T. Cholesterol manufactured in the liver

U. Final, confirmed diagnosis based on clinical signs and symptoms and the results of diagnostic tests

22. Provide the missing information in the plasma flow chart (see Figure 6-1 in the textbook).

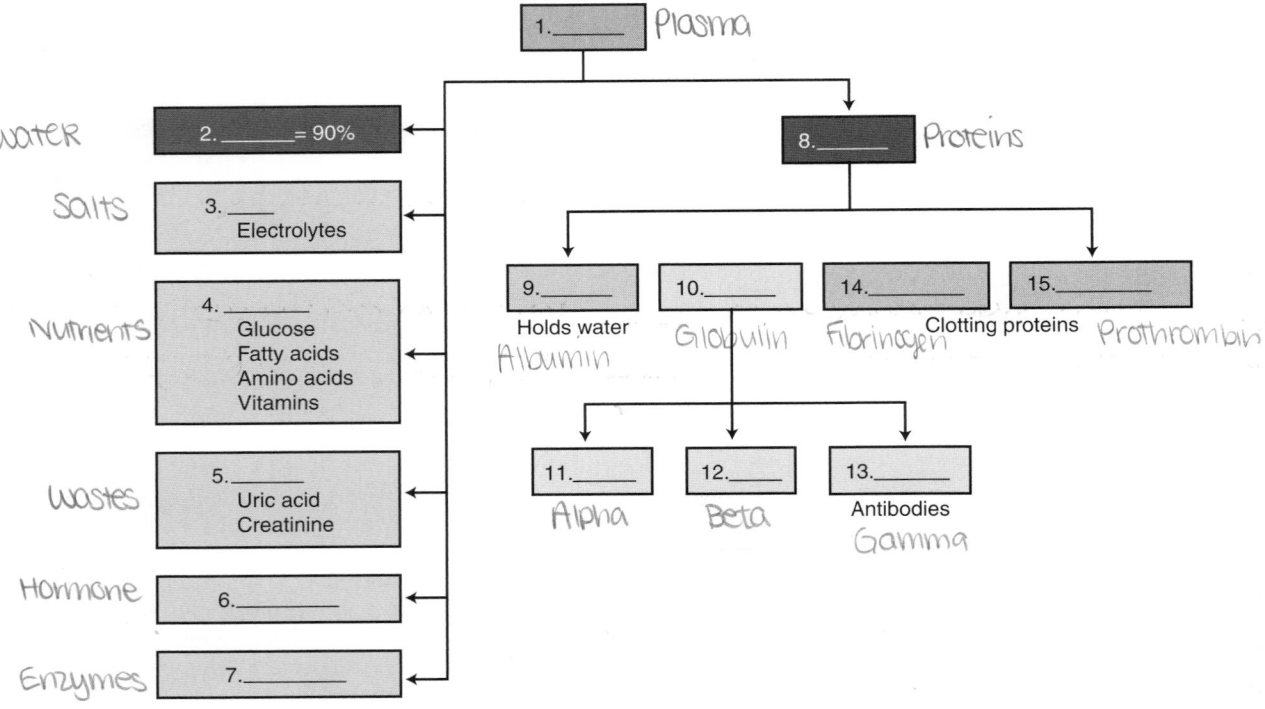

23. Match the categories of chemicals found in plasma with their associated substances (see Figure 6-1 in the textbook).

_____h._____ clotting proteins

_____e._____ nutrients

_____g._____ hormones

_____a._____ proteins

_____i._____ wastes

_____b._____ salts

_____f._____ gamma globulins

_____d._____ enzymes

_____c._____ the three globulins

A. Albumins and globulins
B. Electrolytes
C. Alpha, beta, and gamma
D. Catalysts
E. Glucose, amino acids, and fatty acids
F. Antibodies
G. Thyroid and pituitary glands
H. Prothrombin and fibrinogen
I. Urea, uric acid, creatinine

24. Describe the similarities and differences between the gold "SST" tube and the red "clot" tube.

Red "clot" tube allows the blood to clot with no additives. Gold "SST" tube
yields a serum specimen that is separated from the clot.

Chapter **6** **Chemistry**

pg175

25. Refer to the sample requisition in the textbook (see Figure 6-3), and identify what tube to use for each of the following tests:

prothrombin time	Lt. blue	BUN	Gold
lipid panel	Gold	CBC w/Diff	Purple
renal function panel	Gold	mono test	Red

pg173 26. When prothrombin and fibrinogen are removed from plasma, the remaining liquid is referred to as ___serum___.

27. Define the following glucose-related abbreviations.

A1c ___hemoglobin A1c___

IGT ___impaired glucose tolerance___

FBG ___fasting blood glucose test___

NIDDM ___non-insulin-dependent diabetes mellitus___

FPG ___fasting plasma glucose test___

OGTT ___oral glucose tolerance test___

GTT ___glucose tolerance test___

2-hr PP ___2hr postprandial blood sugar.___

IDDM ___insulin-dependent diabetes mellitus___

pg176 28. How is glucose metabolized in the following locations?

Body cells ___all take in blood glucose for energy___

Liver ___converts excess glucose into glycogen or combines glucose with fatty acids to produce trigly.___

Muscles ___store and convert excess glucose into glycogen.___

Adipose tissue ___take in fatty acids to produce triglycerides.___

pg176 29. List the two ways insulin lowers the level of blood glucose.

___- promoting movement of glucose from blood into body cells___

___- stimulating the conversion of glucose to glycogen in liver and muscles.___

pg176 30. List the two ways glucagon raises the level of blood glucose.

___- stimulating the conversion of the stored glycogen in the liver and muscles back into glucose and then releasing the glucose into blood.___

pg 177 31. What two lifestyle changes can a prediabetic patient make to prevent or delay the development of type 2 diabetes?

___- modest weight loss with diets containing fewer refined carbs.___

___- regular exercise.___

pg180 32. List three beneficial functions of cholesterol.

___- essential for production of cell membrane, bile, myelin sheaths on nerves, and steroid hormones. It's also required in absorption of vitamin D.___

pg181 33. List the two dietary fats that elevate the bad type of cholesterol (LDL).

___- saturated fats___

___- trans fats___

34. Define the following lipid-related abbreviations.

HDL __high-density lipoprotein__

LDL __low-density lipoprotein__

TC/HDL ratio __total cholestrol/high density lipoprotein__

VLDL __very low density lipoprotein__

35. List two dietary fats that elevate the good type of cholesterol (HDL).

   – monounsaturated fats

   – polyunsaturated fats

36. Why is LDL cholesterol referred to as "lousy" cholesterol and HDL referred to as "healthy" cholesterol?

   – lousy (LDL) because it forms plaque on the walls of blood vessels.

   – healthy (HDL) because it has lowest fat content and appears to protect against accumulation of fatty deposits on blood vessels.

37. Physicians are likely to be more interested in which of the following as a predictive indicator of future myocardial infarction?

  a. Cholesterol value

  b. LDL value

  c. Cholesterol/HDL ratio

  d. HDL value

38. People who exercise regularly, maintain normal weight, and eat mostly unsaturated fats will probably increase their level of

  a. HDL

  b. LDL

  c. Albumin

  d. Glucose

39. When testing for triglycerides, the patient should refrain from alcohol for __2__ days before testing and fast for __2-14__ hours before the test.

PROCEDURES: CLINICAL LABORATORY IMPROVEMENT AMENDMENT (CLIA)–WAIVED CHEMISTRY TESTS

40. What is the purpose of *calibrating* a blood chemistry analyzer? (Hint: Think of the calibrator checks when running the Cholestech.)

   It is done to make sure the equipment is working properly.

41. Complete the following tasks.

A. List three reasons or causes why a liquid control would fall outside its designated range.

B. Using the monthly Levy-Jennings chart at the end of this chapter, record the following control settings and daily results for the normal liquid glucose control:

Reference range for control = 96 – 136 mg/dL

+2 standard deviations = 136

+1 standard deviation = 126

Mean = 116

− 1 standard deviation = 106

−2 standard deviations = 96

Daily results:

1. 118	7. 108	13. 137	17. repeat 110	23. 120	29. 114
2. 114	8. 114	13. repeat 125	18. 99	24. 114	30. 115
3. 113	9. 120	14. 117	19. 105	25. 133	31. 116
4. 104	10. 118	15. 106	20. 105	26. 123	
5. 101	11. 120	16. 114	21. 110	27. 130	
6. 100	12. 130	17. 94	22. 118	28. 116	

C. When looking at the chart, were any of the Westgard Rules below broken (circle the numbers that apply)? Should you continue using the monitor and/or strips? _____:

1. Both levels of control results were outside the manufacturer's reference range (if running a normal and high control). *Note:* This rule does not apply because we are monitoring only one control.

2. The same control level fell outside of the reference range in two successive runs.

3. One of the controls fell outside of the plus or minus 1 standard deviation in four successive runs.

4. One of the controls consistently fell above the mean value or consistently fell below the mean value for 10 consecutive runs.

D. (OPTIONAL) If available, chart the class results for the liquid glucose control on the Levy-Jennings chart found in the workbook Appendix, and analyze the results based on the Westgard Rules.

pg184 42. List three foods that the patient should avoid 2 days before collecting a fecal specimen used for the occult blood test.

— Red meat, turnips, horseradish, bananas.

pg196 43. What is the name of home fecal occult blood test for which the patient places the test paper directly into the toilet? _____ If the test area of the paper turns green or blue, is the result positive or negative? _____

ColoCARE method. It is positive.

44. Label the supplies and equipment for the test kit method for A1c (see Procedure 6-2 in the textbook). Which supply item must be used for all 20 tests in the kit? _meter_. May that item be used with cartridges from another kit? _NO_

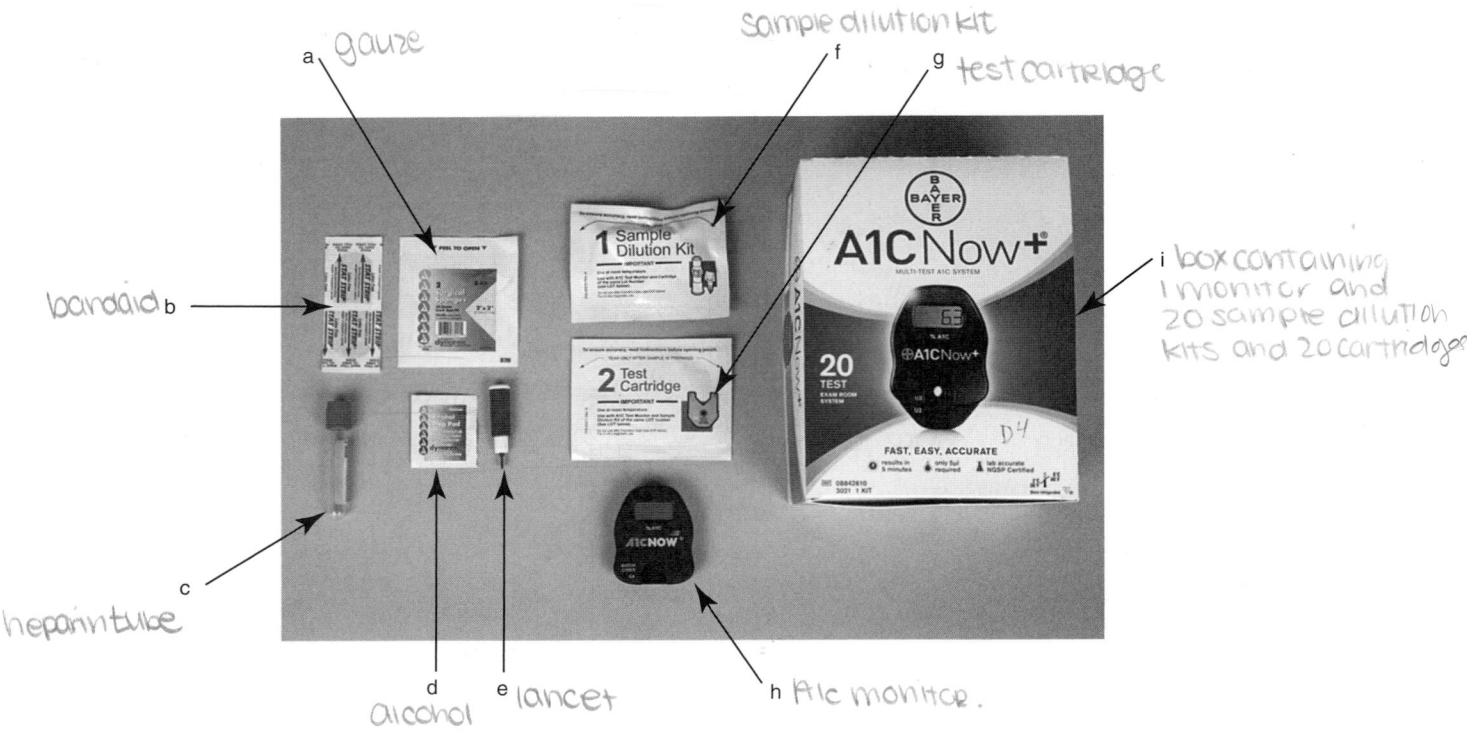

a. gauze
b. bandaid
c. heparin tube
d. alcohol
e. lancet
f. sample dilution kit
g. test cartridge
h. A1c monitor
i. box containing 1 monitor and 20 sample dilution kits and 20 cartridges

45. Label the Cholestech LDX equipment and supplies (see Procedure 6-3 in the textbook).

a. Cholestech LDX analyzer
b. printer with self-adhesive individual report
c. liquid control box with insert reference sheet of values for level 1 + 2 controls.
d. optics check container and cassette for daily optic check.
e. foil wrap and testing cassette
f. capillary tubes + plungers for collecting + dispensing capillary blood samples.

46. Label the ColoScreen III equipment and supplies (see Procedure 6-4 in the textbook).

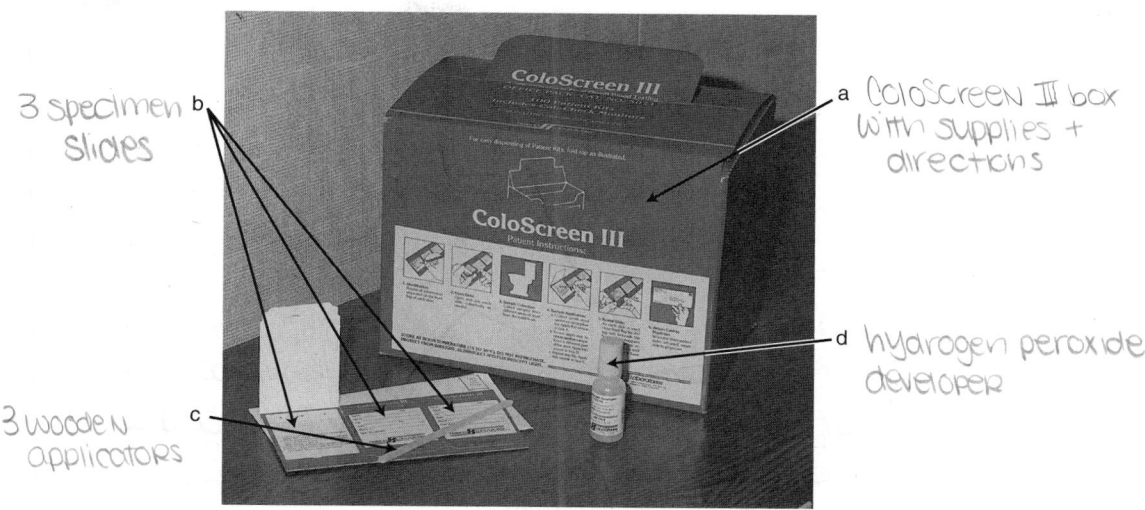

3 specimen b
slides

a ColoScreen III box with supplies + directions

d hydrogen peroxide developer

3 wooden c
applicators

ADVANCED CONCEPTS

Match each procedural and advanced term with the correct definition.

_d._ 47. cation
_m._ 48. galvanometer
_i._ 49. reflectance photometry
_h._ 50. troponins I and T
_k._ 51. bilirubin
_j._ 52. absorbance photometry
_l._ 53. anion
_g._ 54. i-STAT and Piccolo
_f._ 55. transmittance photometry
_e._ 56. calibration
_b._ 57. occult
_a._ 58. gout
_c._ 59. myoglobin

A. Form of arthritis caused by accumulation of uric acid crystals in the synovial fluid
B. Hidden or not visible to the naked eye
C. Heme-containing, oxygen-binding protein found in muscles
D. Positively charged ion
E. "Optics check" or setting to ensure the analyzer's optics are working correctly with the testing devices
F. Measurement of the amount of light passing through the solution
G. CLIA-waived chemistry analyzers
H. Heart-specific indicators of a recent myocardial infarction
I. Measurement of the light that reflects off of the specimen
J. Measurement of the amount of light the solution absorbs
K. Waste product from the breakdown of hemoglobin
L. Negatively charged ion
M. Instrument capable of measuring the intensity of light

60. List eight critical chemistry tests that are typically monitored during a medical emergency:

pH   potassium
PCO$_2$ chloride
PO$_2$ glucose
sodium   Bun

61. Match the panels with their representative group of tests.

_e_ cardiac panel
_d_ hepatic panel
_b_ renal panel
_g_ lipid panel
_f_ thyroid panel
_a_ metabolic panel
_c_ electrolyte panel

A. Twelve or more tests
B. BUN, creatinine, uric acid
C. Sodium, potassium, chloride
D. Bilirubin, AST, ALT, ALP, LD, GGT
E. Troponins I and T, CK, LD, ALT, myoglobin
F. TSH, T_4, T_3 uptake
G. TC, HDL, LDL, triglycerides

✶ 62. Match the analytes with the medical condition or organ that is being monitored.

_e_ uric acid
_d_ cholesterol
_c_ BUN
_a_ glucose
_b_ bilirubin

A. Diabetes
B. Hepatitis or liver function
C. Gout
D. Coronary artery disease and atherosclerosis
E. Nephritis or kidney function

Chemistry Abbreviations

63. Using the alphabetical list of abbreviations at the beginning of Chapter 6 in the textbook, identify the six enzyme abbreviations routinely tested for tissue or organ damage. (Hint: Remember enzymes have the suffix -*ase*.) Then identify two organs or the diseases that are associated with each enzyme. Use the categorical chart of blood chemistry analytes (see Table 6-3 in the textbook) at the end of the chapter to locate the diseases.

Enzyme Abbreviation	Enzyme	Affected Organs and Associated Diseases
1.		
2.		
3.		
4.		
5.		
6.		

64. List the four electrolyte abbreviations found at the beginning of the chapter and state whether they are cations or anions. (Hint: They have positive or negative charges after their abbreviations.)

Electrolyte Abbreviation	Electrolyte	Cation/Anion (+/−)
1.		
2.		
3.		
4.		

Procedure 6-1: Glucometer Procedure

Person evaluated _____ Date _____

Evaluated by _____ Score _____

Outcome goal	To perform FDA-approved CLIA-waived glucose test following the most current OSHA safety guidelines and applying correct quality control
Conditions	Supplies needed: - CONTOUR monitor (previously Ascensia Elite) or One Touch Test Strips - Coded test strip and liquid control - Lancet, alcohol, gauze, bandage - Personal protective equipment
Standards	Required time = 5 minutes Performance time _____ Total possible points = _____ Points earned = _____
Evaluation Rubric Codes: **S** = Satisfactory, meets standard **U** = Unsatisfactory, fails to meet standard	
NOTE: Steps marked with an asterisk (*) are critical to achieve required competency	

Preparation	Scores	
	S	**U**
A. Test information		
- Kit or instrument method: **Contour or One Touch Ultra**		
- Manufacturer: **Bayer or LifeScan**		
- Proper storage (e.g., temperature, light) **test strips and controls are stored at room temperature**		
- Expiration date: _____		
- Lot #: _____ Calibration # _____		
- Package insert or test flow chart available: _____ yes _____ no		
B. Personal protective equipment: **gloves, gown, biohazard container**		
C. Specimen information		
- Type of specimen: **fasting, 2-hour postprandial, or random specimen**		
- Specimen source: **capillary blood or lavender-topped vacuum tube** (Note: gray-topped tubes are not used for this method.)		
- Specimen testing device: **coded test strips**		
D. Assembled all the above, sanitized hands, and applied personal protective equipment.		

Procedure: Analytical Phase	Scores	
	S	U
E. Performed/observed quantitative quality control		
- Calibration check is done automatically when each strip is inserted.		
- (*Note:* Older versions need to set the code number on the meter based on the test strip number,)		
- Control levels: normal _____ high _____		
- (Manufacturer recommendation: Run normal control with each new batch of strips, with each new operator, and then weekly.)		
F. Performed patient test		
1. Turned on meter by inserting test strip's end with the contact bars.		
2. Stuck finger and *touched the end of the strip into the drop* of blood, allowing the blood to flow ("sip") into the strip without interruption.		
- Did **not** smear or place blood on top or bottom of strip.		
3. When beep was heard, removed the glucometer and strip away from drop of blood.		
4. Result displayed on the screen.		
***Accurate Results** _____ **Instructor Confirmation** _____		

Follow-up: Postanalytical Phase	Scores	
	S	U
*G. Proper documentation		
1. On control log: _____ yes _____ no		
2. On patient log: _____ yes _____ no		
3. Documentation on patient chart (see following page)		
H. Identified "critical values" and took appropriate steps to notify physician		
- Expected ranges for glucose based on ADA recommendations		

		Fasting	2-Hour Postprandial (After Drinking a Glucose-Rich Beverage)
	Normal	Less than 100 mg/dL	<140 mg/dL
	Prediabetes	100-125 mg/dL	140-199 mg/dL
	Diabetes	≥126 mg/dL	≥200 mg/dL

	Scores	
I. Proper disposal and disinfection		
1. Disposed all sharps into biohazard sharps containers.		
2. Disposed all other regulated medical waste into biohazard bags.		
3. Disinfected test area and instruments according to OSHA guidelines.		
4. Sanitized hands after removing gloves.		
Total Points per Column		

Patient Name: _____

Patient Chart Entry: (Include when, what, how, why, any additional information, and the signature of the person charting.)

_____

_____

_____

_____

Procedure 6-2: A1c NOW+ Glycosylated Hemoglobin Procedure

Person evaluated _____   Date _____

Evaluated by _____   Score _____

Outcome goal	To perform FDA-approved glycosylated hemoglobin A_{1c} waived test following the most current OSHA safety guidelines and applying the correct quality control
Conditions	Supplies needed: - Gauze, bandage, alcohol swab - Lancet for capillary blood sample or heparin tube with venous blood sample - Sample dilution kit containing capillary tube collector and sampler body - Test cartridge - A_{1c} monitor programmed to work only with the 20 cartridges in the kit - Personal protective equipment
Standards	Required time = 5 minutes Performance time = _____ Total possible points = _____ Points earned = _____

Evaluation Rubric Codes:
S = Satisfactory, meets standard   **U** = Unsatisfactory, fails to meet standard

NOTE: Steps marked with an asterisk (*) are critical to achieve required competency.

Preparation: Preanalytical Phase	Scores	
	S	U
A. Test information		
- Kit or instrument method: **A1c NOW+ test kit method.**		
- Manufacturer: **Bayer.**		
- Proper storage (e.g., temperature, light): **Foil-wrapped cartridges and kits are refrigerated. Allow one hour to warm to room temperature.**		
- Expiration date: _____		
- Lot # of cartridges: _____		
- Package insert or test flow chart available: _____ yes _____ no		
B. Personal protective equipment: **gloves, gown, face shield.**		
C. Proper specimen used for test.		
- Use only **fresh capillary blood** or venous whole blood collected in a **green heparin tube.** Venous blood can be used only if the tube is less than 1 week old and has been refrigerated during that time. Make sure blood in heparin tube is well mixed and at room temperature.		
- Specimen testing device: microcapillary tube provided in kit. After the glass capillary tube has been filled with the specimen, the analysis must begin within 5 minutes.		
D. Assembled all the above and made sure they were at the same temperature (within 18 to 28 degrees Centigrade), sanitized hands, and applied personal protective equipment.		

Procedure: Analytical Phase	Scores	
	S	U
E. Performed/observed quantitative quality control		
- Optics check: Each box of test kits has already set its optics (make sure code on cartridge matches the code on monitor, but do not open until just before inserting into monitor).		
- Control levels: normal _____ abnormal _____		
F. Performed patient test		
1. Removed the blood collector from the foil #1 sampler dilution kit, and gently touched the tip of the capillary tube that was attached to the holder into the small drop of blood from the fingerstick or the venous blood drop on the slide.		
- The blood should fill the small glass capillary tube without touching the plastic holder.		
2. Wiped the sides of the capillary tube with tissue.		
3. Fully inserted the capillary holder into the sampler body that also came from the #1 sampler dilution kit (pushed together and twisted until the holder and sampler body snapped into place).		
4. Mixed sample with the dilution by tilting 6 to 8 times; then stood the sampler on the table.		
5. Opened the #2 test cartridge foil package and performed the following within 2 minutes:		
- Clicked the cartridge into the monitor that came in the same kit box; checked code numbers, which must match		
- While the monitor indicated "WAIT," prepared the sample by removing the base		
- Did not add the sample until the monitor indicated "SMPL"		
- Pushed sampler down onto the white well of the cartridge		
- The monitor was on a level surface and was not moved until the test was complete.		
6. After several minutes, the monitor indicated "QCOK," followed by the test result and by the number of tests left in the kit.		
7. Recorded the results from the display and reported to the physician.		

*Accurate Results _____   Instructor Confirmation _____

Follow-up: Postanalytical Phase	Scores	
	S	U
*G. Proper documentation		
1. Control logs: _____ yes _____ no		
2. Patient log: _____ yes _____ no		
3. Documented on patient chart (see following page).		

4. Identified critical values and took appropriate steps to notify physician.		
- Expected values:		

Nondiabetics	3%-6%
Controlled diabetics	6%-8%
Poorly controlled diabetics	As much as 20% or higher

Note: Because A_{1c} is also affected by the hemoglobin concentration, normal ranges should be determined by each laboratory to conform to the population being tested.

H. Proper disposal and disinfection		
1. Disposed the cartridge into biohazard sharps containers, and returned monitor to the box for subsequent testing.		
2. Disposed all other regulated medical waste into biohazard bags.		
3. Disinfected test area and instruments according to OSHA guidelines.		
4. Sanitized hands after removing gloves.		
Total Points per Column		

Patient Name: _____

Patient Chart Entry: (Include when, what, how, why, any additional information, and the signature of the person charting.)

_____

_____

_____

_____

Procedure 6-3: Cholestech Method of Measuring Lipids and Glucose

Person evaluated _____ Date _____

Evaluated by _____ Score _____

Outcome goal	To perform FDA-approved lipid profile waived test following the most current OSHA safety guidelines and applying the correct quality control.
Conditions	Supplies needed: - Optics check cassette - Level 1 and 2 liquid controls - Alcohol, gauze, and lancets or vacuum lithium heparin tubes - Capillary tubes and plungers for finger stick sample - Mini-Pet pipette and pipette tips for venipuncture sample - Personal protective equipment
Standards	Required time = 10 minutes Performance time = _____ Total possible points = _____ Points earned = _____
Evaluation Rubric Codes: **S** = Satisfactory, meets standard **U** = Unsatisfactory, fails to meet standard	
NOTE: Steps marked with an asterisk (*) are critical to achieve required competency.	

Preparation: Preanalytical Phase	Scores	
	S	**U**
A. Test information		
- Kit or instrument method: **Cholestech LDX Analyzer**		
- Manufacturer: **Cholestech Corporation**		
- Proper storage (e.g., temperature, light): **Foil-wrapped cassettes are refrigerated. They must return to room temperature before testing.**		
- Expiration date: _____		
- Cassette lot #: _____		
- Package insert or test flow chart available: _____ yes _____ no		
B. Personal protective equipment: **gloves, gown, biohazard containers**		
C. Specimen Information		
- Patient preparation: **Fasting recommended for cholesterol. Triglyceride requires fasting and no alcohol consumption in previous 48 hours.**		
- Type of specimen: **capillary blood or lithium heparin (green) tube only for venous blood**		
- Specimen testing device: **Cholestech capillary tube (once in tube, must be tested within 5 minutes)**		
D. Assembled all the above, sanitized hands, and applied personal protective equipment.		

Procedure: Analytical Phase	Scores	
	S	U
E. Performed/observed quantitative quality control		
- Calibration check: **Run calibration cassette daily.**		
- Control levels: **Level 1, Level 2** (Use the mini-Pet pipettes provided by Cholestech)		
F. Performed patient test	**S**	**U**
1. Allowed cassette to come to room temperature (at least 10 minutes before opening).		
2. Made sure analyzer was plugged in and warmed up.		
3. Removed cassette from its pouch and placed it on flat surface.		
- Held cassette by the short sides only.		
- Did not touch the black bar or the brown magnetic strip.		
4. Pressed RUN; the analyzer did a self-test, and the screen displayed "selftest running" and then "selftest OK."		
5. The cassette drawer opened, and the screen displayed "load cassette and press RUN."		
- Drawer remains open for 4 minutes, after which it closes with the message "System timeout: RUN to continue." If the RUN button is not pushed within 15 seconds, the drawer closes, and the screen goes blank. Press RUN again, allow to go through the self-test again, and then proceed.		
6. Collected fresh capillary blood to the black line of the capillary tube with plunger inserted into the red end of the tube.		
- Or collected fresh venous whole blood with the Cholestech mini-Pet pipette.		
7. Placed whole blood sample into the test cassette sample well.		
- The finger stick sample must be put into the cassette within 5 minutes of collection or the blood will clot.		
8. *Immediately* placed cassette into the drawer of the analyzer.		
- Kept cassette level after the sample was applied.		
- The black reaction bar faced toward the analyzer.		
- The brown magnetic strip was on the right.		
9. Pressed RUN. The drawer closed, and the screen displayed "[test names] – running."		
10. When the test was completed, the analyzer beeped, and the screen displayed results at the same time the printer printed results. (Press DATA to display the calculated results of all tests on the screen if running a panel of tests.)		
*Accurate Results _____ Instructor Confirmation _____		

Follow-up: Postanalytical Phase	Scores	
	S	U
*G. Proper documentation		
1. On control log: _____ yes _____ no		

2. On patient log: _____ yes _____ no	
3. Documented on patient chart (see below).	
4. Identified "critical values" and took appropriate steps to notify physician.	

- NCEP ATP III guidelines for lipid panels:

Test	Desirable
Total cholesterol (TC)	<200 mg/dL
HDL cholesterol	>40 mg/dL
LDL cholesterol	<130 mg/dL
Triglycerides	<150 mg/dL
TC/HDL ratio	≤4.5
Glucose	Fasting: 60-110 mg/dL
	Nonfasting: <less than 160 mg/dL
Alanine aminotransferase	10-40 U/L

H. Proper disposal and disinfection		
1. Disposed all sharps into biohazard sharps containers.		
2. Disposed all other regulated medical waste into biohazard bags.		
3. Disinfected test area and instruments according to OSHA guidelines.		
4. Sanitized hands after removing gloves.		
Total Points per Column		

Patient Name: _____

Attach printed readout, or record results on the chart provided:

Test	Results	Desirable
Total cholesterol (TC)		<200 mg/dL
HDL cholesterol		40 mg/dL
LDL cholesterol		<130 mg/dL
Triglycerides		<150 mg/dL
TC/HDL ratio		≤4.5
Other		
Glucose		Fasting: 60-110 mg/dL
		Nonfasting: <160 mg/dL

Procedure 6-4: Occult Blood: ColoScreen III Method

Person evaluated _____ Date _____

Evaluated by _____ Score _____

Outcome goal	To perform FDA-approved, CLIA-waived fecal occult blood test following the most current OSHA safety guidelines and applying the correct quality control
Conditions	Supplies needed: - Three specimen slides - Three wooden applicators - Hydrogen peroxide developer - Personal protective equipment
Standards	Required time = 5 minutes Performance time = _____ Total possible points = _____ Points earned = _____

Evaluation Rubric Codes:
S = Satisfactory, meets standard   **U** = Unsatisfactory, fails to meet standard

NOTE: Steps marked with an asterisk (*) are critical to achieve required competency.

Preparation: Preanalytical Phase	Scores	
	S	**U**
A. Test information		
- Kit or instrument method: **ColoScreen III**		
- Manufacturer: **SmithKline Diagnostics**		
- Proper storage (e.g., temperature, light): **room temperature**		
- Expiration date: _____		
- Lot # on kit: _____		
- Package insert or test flow chart available: _____ yes _____ no		
B. Instructed patient on the following dietary preparations.		
1. Two days before the test and during testing time, the patient should eat a high-fiber diet with any of the following:		
- Well-cooked poultry and fish		
- Cooked fruits and vegetables		
- Bran cereals		
- Raw lettuce, carrots, and celery		
- Moderate amounts of peanuts and popcorn		
2. The patient should avoid ingesting the following substances, which interfere with the test results:		
- Red and partially cooked meats		

	Scores	
	S	U
- Turnips, cauliflower, broccoli, parsnips, and melons (especially cantaloupe)		
- Alcohol, aspirin, and vitamin C		
C. Instructed the patient on how to use the slides, applicators, and the take-home instructions as follows:		
- After a bowel movement, use the wooden applicator to collect a small sample of feces, and spread a thin layer in box A of the slide.		
- Using the same applicator, collect a second sample from a different part of the feces, and spread it in box B.		
- Discard the wooden applicator, reseal the cover of the slide, and complete the information requested on the outside of the cover.		
- Repeat above steps with the remaining applicators for the next two bowel movements and two remaining slides.		

Procedure: Analytical Phase	Scores	
	S	U
D. Personal protective equipment: gloves when testing the slides		
E. Performed occult blood test as follows:		
- Confirmed all necessary information was written on slide covers.		
- Applied gloves and observed universal precautions.		
- Opened the back sides of all three slides and placed two drops of developer on each specimen.		
- Observed slide for 30 seconds to 2 minutes and checked to see if a blue reaction occurred, indicating a positive result.		
F. Performed monitor test (internal control)		
- Placed one or two drops between the monitor boxes and observed for 30 seconds to 2 minutes before reading the results.		
- Confirmed the positive control turned blue and the negative control did not.		

*Accurate Results _____   Instructor Confirmation _____

Follow-up: Postanalytical Phase	Scores	
	S	U
*G. Proper documentation		
1. On control/patient log: _____ yes _____ no		
2. Documented on patient chart (see following page).		
3. Identified critical values and took appropriate steps to notify physician.		
- Expected values for occult blood: negative		
H. Proper disposal and disinfection		
1. Disposed all regulated medical waste into biohazard bags.		
2. Disinfected test area and instruments according to OSHA guidelines.		
3. Sanitized hands after removing gloves.		
Total Points per Column		

Patient Name: _____

Patient Chart Entry: (Include when, what, how, why, any additional information, and the signature of the person charting.)

_____

_____

_____

Procedure 6-5: i-STAT Chemistry Analyzer Procedure

Person evaluated _____ Date _____

Evaluated by _____ Score _____

Outcome goal	To perform FDA-approved i-STAT chemistry waived test following the most current OSHA safety guidelines and applying the correct quality control
Conditions	Supplies needed: - i-STAT 1 handheld, recharging dock, and printer - Ampule of Level 1 liquid control for i-STAT CHEM 8+ - i-STAT CHEM 8+ cartridges - Fresh blood collected in lithium heparin tubes (green top) - 1-mL plain syringe - Safety transfer device or safety tip - Personal protective equipment and biohazard container
Standards	Required time = 15 minutes Performance time = _____ Total possible points = _____ Points earned _____
Evaluation Rubric Codes: **S** = Satisfactory, meets standard **U** = Unsatisfactory, fails to meet standard	
NOTE: Steps marked with an asterisk (*) are critical to achieve required competency.	

Preparation: Preanalytical Phase	Scores	
	S	**U**
A. Test information		
- Kit or instrument method: **i-STAT Chemistry Analyzer**		
- Manufacturer: **Abbott**		
- Proper storage (e.g., temperature, light): **Foil-wrapped cartridges and controls are refrigerated. They must return to room temperature before testing.**		
- Expiration date: _____		
- Scan cartridge lot #: _____		
- Package insert or test flow chart available: _____ yes _____ no		
B. Personal protective equipment: **gloves, gown, biohazard containers**		
C. Specimen information		
- Patient preparation: **Collect blood, making sure the 4-mL heparin tube fills completely and is mixed by tilting 10 times. Specimen should be tested within 10 minutes.**		
- Type of specimen: **Lithium heparin (green) tube only for venous blood**		
- Specimen testing device: **A 1-mL syringe is used to remove the specimen from the green vacuum tube and transfer the blood to the cartridge.**		
D. Assembled all the above, sanitized hands, and applied personal protective equipment.		

Procedure: Analytical Phase	Scores	
	S	U
E. Performed/observed quantitative quality control		
- Calibration check: **Use the simulator provided by i-STAT.**		
- Control level: **Level 1 ampule is provided by i-STAT.**		
F. Performed patient test	S	U
1. Allowed cassette to come to room temperature (at least 10 minutes before opening).		
2. Keyed in operator and patient information into the handheld analyzer, followed by scanning the cartridge bar code until a beep was heard.		
3. *Within 10 minutes* of drawing a 4-mL specimen of blood into a vacuum tube, performed the following:		
- Mixed the specimen by tilting 10 times.		
- Connected a safety tip or safety transfer device to a 1-mL syringe.		
- Inverted the green-top tube with the specimen and pierced the green stopper with the syringe safety tip or the transfer device.		
- *Slowly* pulled back on the syringe plunger until it was about one-half full; noted any air bubbles that entered syringe while transferring and did not push them back into specimen.		
- Disconnected syringe from vacuum tube and continued to hold it with tip pointed upward; then held a gauze pad at tip to absorb blood while syringe plunger slowly pushed out the air and approximately three drops of blood.		
- Tore open the foiled cartridge pouch and removed the cartridge by holding the sides and placed it on a flat surface.		
- Held the syringe tip directly over sample well and carefully pushed the blood into the cartridge until the blood reached the arrow and there was still blood remaining in the well but not overflowing.		
4. Moved the tab over the well from left to right using one finger; did not press on the beige circle area directly over the well; pushed down on the tab until it snapped into place.		
5. Used the grooved area to the left of the well or the sides of the cartridge to slowly insert it into the analyzer.		
- The handheld first displayed "Identifying Cartridge" and then a time-to-result bar.		
- ***Did not*** **remove cartridge until the "Cartridge Locked" message was removed and results were displayed on screen.**		
6. Review results		
- After 2 to 3 minutes, the results appeared on the screen. The "→ Page" command on bottom of the screen indicated more results would appear on a second screen. Pressed the print button to send the results to the printer by wireless transmission or by the docking device USB connection.		
The handheld showed the numerical values and units with the results. It also showed bar graphs with tic marks for reference ranges.		
*Accurate Results _____ **Instructor Confirmation** _____		

Follow-up: Postanalytical Phase	Scores	
	S	U
*G. Proper documentation		
1. On control log: _____ yes _____ no		
2. On patient log: _____ yes _____ no		
3. Documented on patient chart (see below).		
4. Identified "critical values" and took appropriate steps to notify physician.		
*SEE TABLE OF TEST RANGES BELOW.		
H. Proper disposal and disinfection		
1. Disposed all sharps into biohazard sharps containers.		
2. Disposed all other regulated medical waste into biohazard bags.		
3. Disinfected test area and instruments according to OSHA guidelines.		
4. Sanitized hands after removing gloves.		
Total Points per Column		

Test	Test Symbol	Units	Reportable Range	Reference Range	Critical Low	Critical High
Sodium	Na	mmol/L	100-180	138-146		
Potassium	K	mmol/L	2.0-9.0	3.5-4.9		
Chloride	Cl	mmol/L	65-140	98-109		
Total carbon dioxide	TCO_2	mmol/L	5-50	24-29		
Ionized calcium	iCa	mmol/L	0.25-2.50	1.12-1.32		
Glucose	Glu	mg/dL	20-700	70-105		
Urea nitrogen	BUN	mg/dL	3-140	8-26		
Creatinine	Crea	mg/dL	0.2-20.0	0.6-1.3		
Hematocrit	Hct	% PCV	10-75	38-51		
Hemoglobin*	Hb	g/dL	3.4-25.5	12-17		
Anion gap*	AnGap	mmol/L	10-99	10-20		

Patient Name: _____

Attach printed readout, or record results on the chart provided:

Test	Test Symbol	Results
Sodium	Na	
Potassium	K	
Chloride	Cl	
Total carbon dioxide	TCO$_2$	
Ionized calcium	iCa	
Glucose	Glu	
Urea nitrogen	BUN	
Creatinine	Crea	
Hematocrit	Hct	
Hemoglobin*	Hb	
Anion Gap*	AnGap	

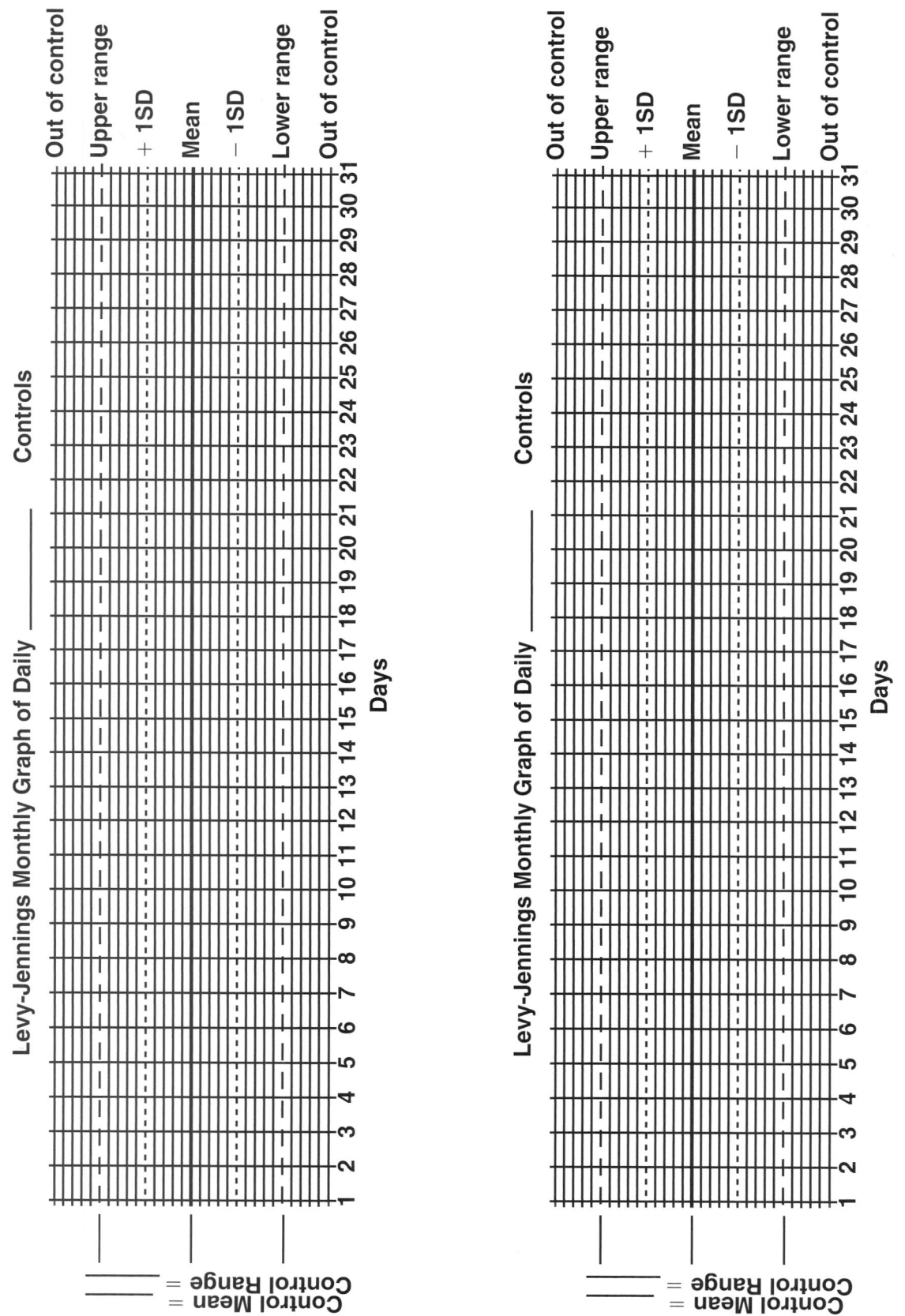

Levy-Jennings Monthly Graph of Daily Controls

7 Immunology

VOCABULARY REVIEW

Match each term with the correct definition.

A. active immunity   G. histamine   M. normal flora

B. autoimmune diseases   H. humoral immunity   N. passive immunity

C. antibodies   I. inflammation   O. phagocytes

D. antigens   J. interferons   P. phagocytosis

E. cell-mediated immunity   K. mucous membrane

F. complement proteins   L. natural killer cells

___h.___ 1. B lymphocytic cell response to antigens resulting in the production of specific antibodies to destroy a foreign invader; also called antibody-mediated immunity

___o.___ 2. Cells capable of engulfing and ingesting microorganisms and cellular debris

___g.___ 3. Compound released by injured cells that causes the dilation of blood vessels

___c.___ 4. Immunoglobulins produced specifically to destroy foreign invaders

___a.___ 5. Long-term protection against future infections resulting from the production of antibodies formed naturally during an infection or artificially by vaccination

___m.___ 6. Nonpathogenic microorganisms that normally inhabit the skin and mucous membranes

___i.___ 7. Overall reaction of the body to tissue injury or invasion by an infectious agent; characterized by redness, heat, swelling, and pain

___p.___ 8. Process of engulfing and digesting microorganisms and cellular debris

___j.___ 9. Proteins secreted by infected cells to prevent the further replication and spread of an infection into neighboring cells

___f.___ 10. Proteins that stimulate phagocytosis and inflammation and are capable of destroying bacteria

___N.___ 11. Short-term acquired immunity created by antibodies received naturally through the placenta (or the colostrum to an infant) or artificially by injection

___l.___ 12. Special type of lymphocyte that attacks and destroys infected cells and cancer cells in a nonspecific way

___d.___ 13. Substances that are perceived as foreign to the body and elicit an antibody response

___e.___ 14. T-lymphocytic cell response to antigens

___k.___ 15. Thin sheets of tissue that line the internal cavities and canals of the body and serve as a barrier against the entry of pathogens

___b.___ 16. Destructive tissue diseases caused by antibody/self-antigen reactions

Match the B and T lymphocytes with their functions.

A. killer T cells   D. helper T cells (T$_H$4 or CD4)

B. suppressor T cells   E. memory B cells

C. plasma cells   F. memory T cells

_____e_____ 17. Antigen-activated B lymphocytes that remember an identified antigen for future encounters

_____a_____ 18. Antigen-activated lymphocytes that attack foreign antigens directly and destroy cells that bear the antigens; also called cytotoxic cells

_____b_____ 19. Antigen-activated lymphocytes that inhibit T and B cells after enough cells have been activated

_____d_____ 20. Antigen-activated lymphocytes that stimulate other T cells and help B cells produce antibodies

_____f_____ 21. Antigen-activated T lymphocytes that remember an antigen for future encounters

_____c_____ 22. Subgroup of B lymphocytes that produce the antibodies that travel through the blood specifically targeting and reacting with antigens

Match the immunology testing and disease terms with the correct definition.

A. agglutination	E. immunosorbent	I. serology
B. chromatographic	F. in vitro	J. titer
C. erythroblastosis fetalis	G. in vivo	K. vaccination
D. heterophile antibody	H. self-antigens	L. wheal

_____d_____ 23. Antibody that appears during an Epstein-Barr viral infection (mononucleosis) that has an unusual affinity to heterophile antigens on sheep red cells

_____i_____ 24. Branch of laboratory medicine that performs antibody/antigen testing with serum

_____a_____ 25. Clumping together of blood cells or latex beads caused by antibodies adhering to their antigens

_____c_____ 26. A hemolytic anemia in newborns resulting from maternal-fetal blood group incompatibility

_____f_____ 27. Testing in a laboratory apparatus

_____b_____ 28. Pertaining to a visual color change that appears when an enzyme-linked antibody/antigen reaction occurs

_____e_____ 29. Pertaining to the attachment of an antigen or antibody to a solid surface such as latex beads, wells in plastic dishes, or plastic cartridges

_____k_____ 30. Process of injecting harmless or killed microorganisms into the body to induce immunity against a potential pathogen; also called immunization

_____L_____ 31. Raised induration

_____h_____ 32. Substances within the body that induce the production of antibodies that attack an individual's own body tissues; also called autoantigens

_____j_____ 33. A quantitative test that measures the amount of antibody that reacts with a specific antigen

_____g_____ 34. Testing within a host or living organism

FUNDAMENTAL CONCEPTS

pg 210-211 35. When a pathogen is invading the body, list two examples of protection for each line of defense:

First line of external defenses: Skin and mucous membranes

Second line of internal, nonspecific defenses: Phagocytes and natural killer cells.

Third line of internal, specific defenses: T cells and B cells.

pg 211 36. List two white cells that are phagocytic.

Neutrophils and monocytes.

pg 211 37. Give an example of a normal flora organism, and describe how it prevents the invasion of pathogens.

In respiratory tract the mucous membranes contains mucus, which entraps foreign organisms.

pg 212 38. List the clinical signs of inflammation.

Heat, Redness, swelling, and pain

pg 210-212 39. Describe antigens.

Its a substances that are preceived as foreign to the body. Once antibodies are produced, they attack the antigens, forming an antibody/antigen complex that destroys or renders invader harmless.

pg 212 40. Which cells are associated with cell-mediated immunity?

T cells and small lymphocytes

pg 210 41. What is another name for antibodies? (Hint: They are a subcategory of proteins.)

immunoglobulins

pg 213 42. Name the five types of antibodies by their immunoglobulin identification.

IgE, IgM, IgG, IgA, IgD

pg 214 43. Refer to Figure 7-4A and B in the textbook and give examples of natural and artificial active immunity and natural and artificial passive immunity.

Natural active immunity contract disease and produce memory cells
Artificial active immunity recieve a vaccination and produce memory cells.
Natural passive immunity recieve maternal antibodies through placenta/breast milk.
Artificial passive immunity recieve antiserum with antibodies from another host.

44. The pregnancy test determines the presence of what antigenic substance?

    human chorionic gonadotropin

45. Fill in the blanks for the following medical information regarding infectious mononucleosis:

    Causative agent: _Epstein-Barr virus. (kissing disease)_

    Clinical symptoms: _mental and physical fatigue, severe weakness, headache, fever, sore throat, swollen lymph nodes_

    Hematology findings: _increase in reactive lymphocytes._

    Immunology findings: _the antibody that is produced during EBV infection heterophile antibody._

46. Label the QuickVue+ infectious mononucleosis supplies (see Procedure 7-2 in the textbook).

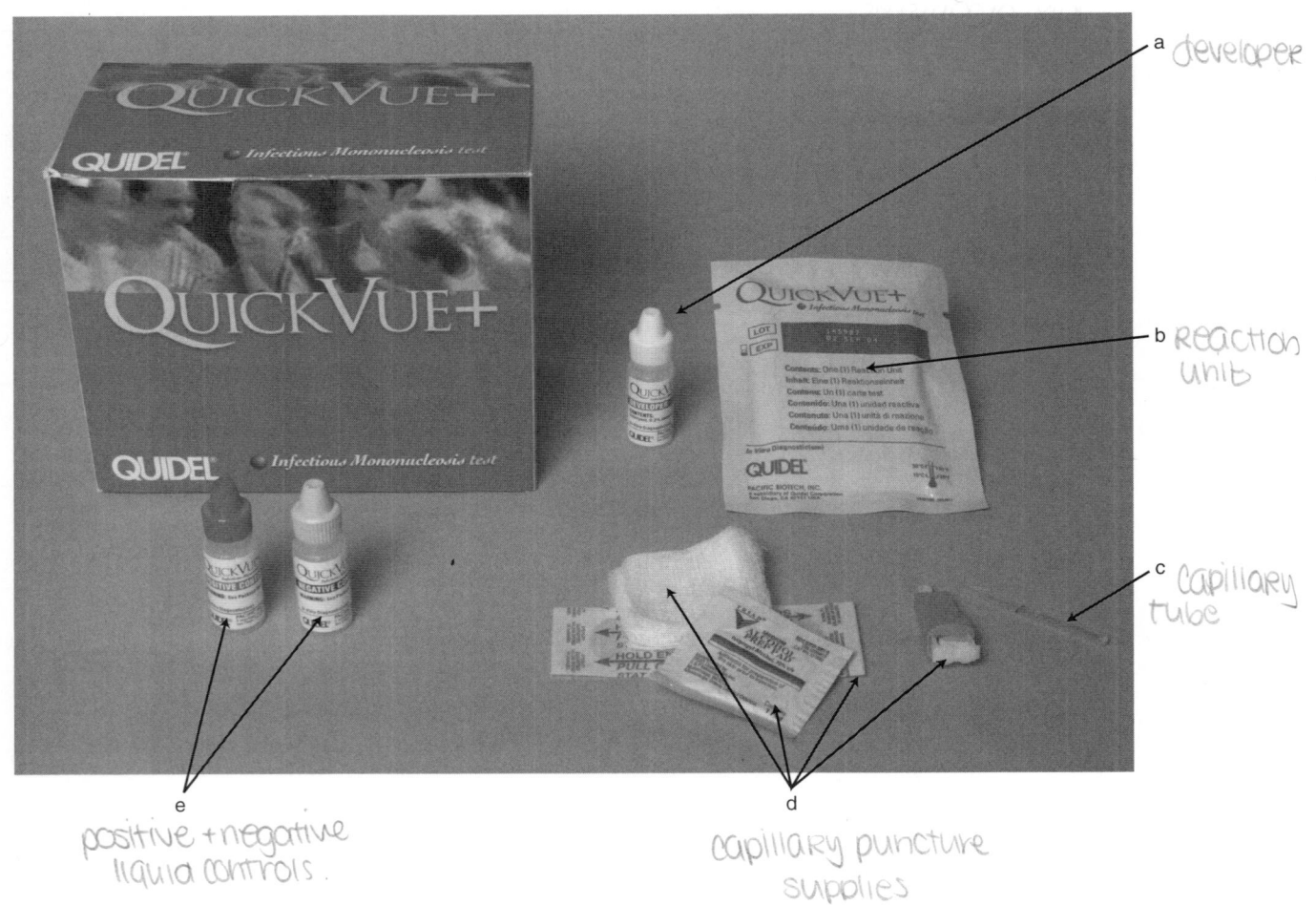

a _developer_

b _reaction unit_

c _capillary tube_

d _capillary puncture supplies_

e _positive + negative liquid controls._

47. Describe the relation between *Helicobacter pylori* and ulcers.

It is a spiral-shaped bacteria that is believed to be the cause of most peptic ulcers (90% of duodenal and 80% of gastric ulcers)

48. Label the QuickVue *H. pylori* supplies (see Procedure 7-3 in the textbook).

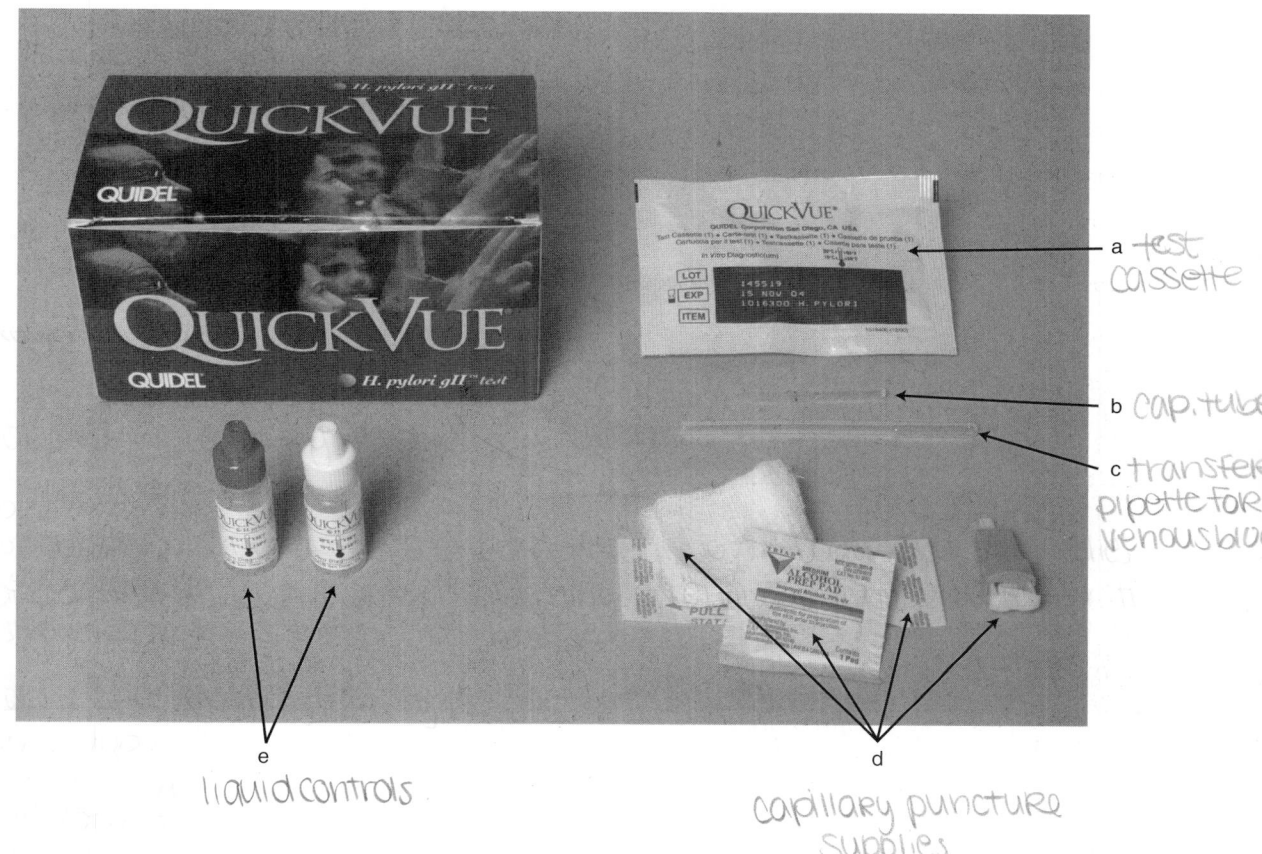

a test cassette

b cap. tube

c transfer pipette for venous blood

e liquid controls

d capillary puncture supplies

49. Based on the test results illustrated in the chart, interpret the results for each test as negative, positive, or invalid.

	Test	Figure in Textbook	Interpreted Result
A		Figure 7-6	-negative REACTION in test aREa and positive Reaction.
B		Procedure 7-1B	-positive REactions in test aRea and control aRea.
C		Procedure 7-2D	-negative RESult and "test complete" Result

50. List three methods for testing for fecal occult blood. (Hint: Two methods are in Chapter 6, and one is in Chapter 7.)

- ColoScreen III
- ColoCare
- iFOB Kits

ADVANCED CONCEPTS

51. Define agglutination.

   — is the visible clumping together of blood cells or other particulate matter such as latex beads.

52. Define immunohematology, and give three reasons why testing is done in this area.

   (blood bank) It is to determine blood types for transfusions, paternity determinations, mother/baby blood compatibility, and forensic investigations

53. Name the blood type for a person who has the following: A and D antigens on red blood cells and anti-B antibodies in the serum.

   A+

54. Name the antigens and antibodies found in type AB blood.

   Antigens (A and B) antibodies (no antibodies)

55. Identify the following ABO blood types based on their agglutination reactions with anti-A and anti-B sera. (Hint: See Procedure 7-4 in the textbook.)

Blood Type		Reaction with Anti-A and Anti-B
AB		Anti-A serum Anti-B serum
B		
O		
A		

56. Identify which of the following is Rh positive and which is Rh negative. (Hint: See Procedure 7-4 in the textbook.)

Rh Type	Reaction with Rh (anti-D) on the Left and the Negative Control on the Right
_Rh−_	
_Rh+_	

57. When the body is exposed to the following pathogens, it produces specific antibodies that can be measured in the plasma or serum. Refer to Table 7-3 in the textbook, and identify the following pathogenic diseases and indicate whether the pathogen is a bacteria or virus.

Pathogen	Disease	Bacteria or Virus
RSV	bronchiolitis / pheumonia	virus
Rubella	birth defect in Fetus	virus
Chlamydia	sexual transmitted disease	Bacterial
Varicella zoster	herpes zoster	virus
B. burgdorferi	lyme diseas	Bacterial

58. List three cancers that can be detected by immunologic testing (see Table 7-3 in the textbook).

Syphilis, varicella zoster, Rheumatoid factor.

Procedure 7-1: SureStep Pregnancy Test Procedure

Person evaluated _____   Date _____

Evaluated by _____   Score _____

Outcome goal	To perform FDA-approved, CLIA-waived urine pregnancy test following the most current OSHA safety guidelines and applying the correct quality control

Conditions	Supplies required:
	- SureStep test kit containing
	  - Individually wrapped test devices
	  - Disposal dropper pipettes
	  - Instruction insert
	- Other materials needed
	  - Urine collection container
	  - Timer
	  - Liquid positive and negative controls for human chorionic gonadotropin (hCG)

Standards	Required time = 5 minutes Performance time = _____ Total possible points = _____ Points earned = _____
Evaluation Rubric Codes: **S** = Satisfactory, meets standard **U** = Unsatisfactory, fails to meet standard	
NOTE: Steps marked with an asterisk (*) are critical to achieve required competency.	

SureStep Pregnancy Test	Scores	
Preparation: Preanalytical Phase	**S**	**U**
A. Test information		
- Kit method: **SureStep**		
- Manufacturer: **Applied Biotech, Inc.**		
- Proper storage (e.g., temperature, light): **refrigerator or room temperature**		
- Lot # of kit: _____		
- Expiration date: _____		
- Package insert or test flow chart available: _____ yes _____ no		
B. Personal protective equipment: **gloves, gown, biohazard container**		
C. Specimen information: **clear urine specimen (centrifuge if cloudy)**		
- Type of specimen: **Preferably first morning urine specimen. Urine can be stored in refrigerator for up to 72 hours but must be tested at room temperature.**		
- Appropriate container: **clean, dry, plastic or glass container**		

Procedure for SureStep hCG: Analytical Phase	Scores	
	S	U
D. Performed/observed qualitative quality control		
- External liquid controls: positive _____ negative _____		
- Internal control: **Colored band appears in the control region (C).**		
E. Performed patient test	S	U
1. Sanitized hands and applied gloves.		
2. Removed test device from its protective pouch and labeled with patient identification.		
- Brought to room temperature before opening to avoid condensation.		
3. Drew up the urine sample to the line marked on the pipette provided in kit.		
- Approximately 0.2 mL		
- Used separate pipettes and devices for each specimen and control.		
4. Dispensed entire contents into the sample well.		
5. Waited for pink-colored bands to appear.		
- High concentrations of hCG can be observed in as little as 40 seconds.		
- Low concentrations may need 4 minutes for the reaction time.		
- Did not interpret results after 10 minutes.		
6. At 5 minutes, read and recorded the results (circled result).		
- Positive = Two distinct pink bands appear, one in the patient test region (T) and one in the control region (C).		
- Negative = Only one pink band appears in the control region (C); no apparent pink band appears in the patient test region (T).		
- Invalid = a total absence of pink bands in control region; test must be repeated with a new device. If problem persisted, called for assistance.		
*Accurate Results _____ **Instructor Confirmation _____**		
Follow-up: Postanalytical	Scores	
	S	U
*F. Proper documentation		
1. On control/patient log: _____ yes _____ no		
2. Documented on patient chart (see following page).		
3. Identified critical values and took appropriate steps to notify physician.		
- Expected values for analyte: negative for pregnancy		

G. Proper disposal and disinfection		
1. Disposed all sharps into biohazard sharps containers.		
2. Disposed all other regulated medical waste into biohazard bags.		
3. Disinfected test area and instruments according to OSHA guidelines.		
Total Points per Column		

Patient Name: _____

Patient Chart Entry: (Include when, what, how, why, any additional information, and the signature of the person charting.)

_____

_____

_____

Procedure 7-2: QuickVue+ Mononucleosis Test Procedure

Person evaluated _____   Date _____

Evaluated by _____   Score _____

Outcome goal	To perform FDA-approved, CLIA-waived infectious mononucleosis test following the most current OSHA safety guidelines and applying the correct quality control

Conditions	Supplies required:
	- QuickVue test kit containing:
	   - Developer
	   - Individually wrapped reaction units
	   - Capillary tubes for capillary blood and pipettes for venous blood
	   - Positive and negative liquid controls
	   - Instruction insert and pictorial flow chart
	- Other materials needed
	   - Capillary puncture supplies (lancet, alcohol, gauze, bandage), or whole blood venipuncture specimen
	   - Timer
	   - Personal protective equipment

Standards	Required time = 10 minutes Performance time = _____ Total possible points = _____ Points earned = _____
Evaluation Rubric Codes: **S** = Satisfactory, meets standard **U** = Unsatisfactory, fails to meet standard	
NOTE: Steps marked with an asterisk (*) are critical to achieve required competency.	

Preparation for Mononucleosis Test: Preanalytical Phase	Scores	
	S	**U**
A. Test information		
- Kit method: **QuickVue+ Mononucleosis Test**		
- Manufacturer: **Quidel**		
- Proper storage (e.g., temperature, light): **room temperature**		
- Lot # of kit: _____		
- Expiration date: _____		
- Package insert or test flow chart available _____ yes _____ no		
B. Personal protective equipment: **gloves, gown, biohazard containers**		
C. Specimen information		
- Use the capillary transfer tube provided in the kit to obtain capillary blood or the larger transfer pipette in the kit to obtain the venipuncture whole blood and the liquid controls.		

Procedure for Mononucleosis: Analytical Phase	Scores	
	S	U
D. Performed/observed qualitative quality control		
- External liquid controls: positive _____ negative _____		
- Internal control: **The color blue fills the "read result" window.**		
E. Performed patient test	S	U
1. Dispensed all the blood from the capillary tube into the "add" well or transferred a large drop from the venous whole blood specimen with the pipette.		
2. Added five drops of developer to the "add" well.		
- Held bottle vertical and allowed drops to fall freely.		
3. Read results at 5 minutes.		
- "Test complete" line must be visible by 10 minutes.		
4. Interpretation of results (circled result):		
- Positive = Any shade of a blue vertical line forms a positive (+) sign in the "read result" window along with the blue "test complete" line. Even a faint blue vertical line should be reported as a positive result.		
- Negative = No blue vertical line appears in the "read result" window along with the blue "test complete" line.		
- Invalid = After 10 minutes, no signal is observed in the "test complete" window, or the color blue fills the "read result" window. If either occurs, the test must be repeated with a new reaction unit. If the problem continues, contact technical support.		
*Accurate Results _____ Instructor Confirmation _____		

Follow-up: Postanalytical Phase	Scores	
	S	U
*F. Proper documentation		
1. On control/patient log: _____ yes _____ no		
2. Documented on patient chart (see following page).		
3. Identified critical values and took appropriate steps to notify physician.		
- Expected values for analyte: negative for mononucleosis		

G. Proper disposal and disinfection		
1. Disposed all sharps into biohazard sharps containers.		
2. Disposed all other regulated medical waste into biohazard bags.		
3. Disinfected test area and instruments according to OSHA guidelines.		
4. Sanitized hands after removing gloves.		
Total Points per Column		

Patient Name: _____

Patient Chart Entry: (Include when, what, how, why, any additional information, and the signature of the person charting.)

_____

_____

_____

Procedure 7-3: QuickVue *Helicobacter pylori* gII Test (CLIA-Waived) Procedure

Person evaluated _____   Date _____

Evaluated by _____   Score _____

Outcome goal	To perform a CLIA-waived *H. pylori* test following the most current OSHA safety guidelines and applying the correct quality controls

Conditions	Supplies required:
	- QuickVue *H. pylori* test kit containing
	  - Foil-wrapped test cassettes
	  - Plastic capillary tubes for fingerstick blood
	  - Disposable droppers for venous blood
	  - Liquid controls: positive and negative external controls
	  - Direction insert and procedure card
	- Other materials needed
	  - Capillary puncture supplies (lancet, alcohol, gauze, bandage) or whole blood venipuncture specimen
	  - Timer
	  - Personal protective equipment

Standards	Required time = 10 minutes Performance time = _____ Total possible points = _____ Points earned = _____
Evaluation Rubric Codes: **S** = Satisfactory, meets standard **U** = Unsatisfactory, fails to meet standard	
NOTE: Steps marked with an asterisk (*) are critical to achieve required competency.	

Preparation for *H. pylori* Test: Preanalytical Phase	Scores	
	S	**U**
A. Test information		
- Kit method: **QuickVue *H. pylori* gII test**		
- Manufacturer: **Quidel**		
- Proper storage of kit: **room temperature**		
- Lot # of kit: _____		
- Expiration date: _____		
- Package insert or test flow chart available: _____ yes _____ no		
B. Personal protective equipment: gloves, gown, biohazard containers		
C. Specimen information		
- Use the capillary tube provided in the kit to obtain capillary blood or the larger disposable dropper in the kit to obtain the venipuncture whole blood specimen and the liquid controls.		

Procedure for *H. pylori*: Analytical Phase	Scores	
	S	**U**
D. Performed/observed qualitative quality control		
- External liquid controls: positive _____ negative _____		
- Internal control: **a blue band of color near the letter C**		

	S	U
E. Performed patient test		
1. Dispensed the blood into the sample well by one of the following methods:		
- Transferred a large drop from the venous anticoagulated whole blood specimen with the disposable dropper.		
- Dispensed all the finger stick blood from the capillary tube.		
- Added two hanging drops of whole blood directly from a finger stick into the round sample well on the test cassette.		
2. Read and recorded results at 5 minutes.		
- Did not move the test cassette until the assay was complete.		
- Some positive results may be seen earlier than 5 minutes.		
3. Interpretation of results (circle result).		
- Positive = a pink line next to the letter T and a blue line next to the letter C		
- Negative = only a blue line next to the letter C		
- Invalid = no blue line next to the letter C; the test must be repeated with a new cassette. If the problem continues, contact technical support.		
*Accurate Results _____ Instructor Confirmation _____		

	Scores	
Follow-up: Postanalytical	S	U
*F. Proper documentation		
1. On control/patient log: _____ yes _____ no		
2. Documented on patient chart (see below).		
3. Identified critical values and took appropriate steps to notify physician		
- Expected values for analyte: negative for *H. pylori*		
G. Proper disposal and disinfection		
1. Disposed all sharps into biohazard sharps containers.		
2. Disposed all other regulated medical waste into biohazard bags.		
3. Disinfected test area and instruments according to OSHA guidelines.		
4. Sanitized hands after removing gloves.		
Total Points per Column		

Patient Name: _____

Patient Chart Entry: (Include when, what, how, why, any additional information, and the signature of the person charting.)

_____

_____

_____

GENERIC ANALYTICAL TEST FORM (FOR KITS NOT COVERED IN THE TEXTBOOK OR WORKBOOK)

Qualitative Test: _____

Person evaluated _____   Date _____

Evaluated by _____   Score _____

Outcome goal	
Conditions	Supplies required:
Standards	Required time = Performance time = _____ Total possible points = _____ Points earned = _____
Evaluation Rubric Codes: **S** = Satisfactory, meets standard **U** = Unsatisfactory, fails to meet standard	
NOTE: Steps marked with an asterisk (*) are critical to achieve required competency.	

Preparation: Preanalytical Phase	Scores	
	S	**U**
A. Test information		
- Kit method:		
- Manufacturer:		
- Proper storage (e.g., temperature, light):		
- Lot # of kit: _____		
- Expiration date: _____		
- Package insert or test flow chart available _____ yes _____ no		
B. Personal protective equipment:		
C. Specimen information:		

Procedure: Analytical Phase	Scores	
	S	**U**
D. Performed/observed qualitative quality control		
- External liquid controls: positive _____ negative _____		
- Internal control		
E. Performed patient test		
1.		
2.		
3.		

	Scores	
4.		
Positive =		
Negative =		
Invalid =		
*Accurate Results _____ Instructor Confirmation _____		

Follow-up: Postanalytical Phase	Scores	
	S	U
*F. Proper documentation		
1. On control/patient log: _____ yes _____ no		
2. Documented on patient chart (see below).		
3. Identified positive values and took appropriate steps to notify physician.		
G. Proper disposal and disinfection		
1. Disposed all sharps into biohazard sharps containers.		
2. Disposed all other regulated medical waste into biohazard bags.		
3. Disinfected test area and instruments according to OSHA guidelines.		
4. Sanitized hands after removing gloves.		
Total Points per Column		

Patient Name: _____

Patient Chart Entry: (Include when, what, how, why, any additional information, and the signature of the person charting.)

_____

_____

_____

8 Microbiology

VOCABULARY REVIEW

Match each definition with the correct term.

_i_   1. malaise

_c_   2. myalgia

_g_   3. expectoration

_e_   4. gram positive

_j_   5. fastidious

_l_   6. mortality

_b_   7. gram negative

_f_   8. infection

_h_   9. peptidoglycan

_a_   10. morbidity

_k_   11. eukaryotic

_d_   12. prokaryote

_m_   13. binary fission

A. Rate at which illness occurs
B. Having the pink or red color of the counterstain used in Gram's method of staining microorganisms
C. Diffuse muscle pain
D. Pertaining to unicellular organisms that do not have a true nucleus with a nuclear membrane
E. Retaining the purple color of the stain used in Gram's method of staining microorganisms
F. Disease in the body caused by the invasion of pathogenic microorganisms
G. Coughing up sputum and mucus from the trachea and lungs
H. Component made of polysaccharides and peptides that gives rigidity to the bacterial cell wall
I. Feeling of weakness, distress, or discomfort
J. Requiring special nutrients for growth
K. Pertaining to organisms that possess a true nucleus with a nuclear membrane and organelles
L. Rate of deaths
M. Asexual reproduction in which the cell splits in half

FUNDAMENTAL CONCEPTS

14. Give an example of an organism that is normal flora, and discuss what can occur if the organism is destroyed.

Lactobacillus in a female vagina. Certain antibiotics destroy Lactobacillus thereby allowing opportunistic infections such as yeast infections.

15. Using Table 8-1 in the textbook, list two health issues of concern in the 1990s.

Multidrug resistance, Rise of tuberculosis, shorter hospital stays, the overuse of antibiotics, and new diseases such as Hantavirus and Ebola virus.

16. List two characteristics of bacteria.

Coccus, Bacillus, and spirillum

17. Explain the difference between a yeast fungus and a mold fungus.

Yeasts are single cells that reproduce by budding, in which a new cell forms on the surface of the yeast, grows, pinches off, and becomes separate cell. Molds are made up of mycelium which consists of tubelike structures called hyphae.

18. List the three general types of bacterial shapes, and give an example of each.

Coccus is Round bacteria. Bacillus is Rod-Shaped bacteria. Spirillum is spiral-shaped bacteria.

19. Match each bacterial shape or group with its name (see Figure 8-1 in the textbook).

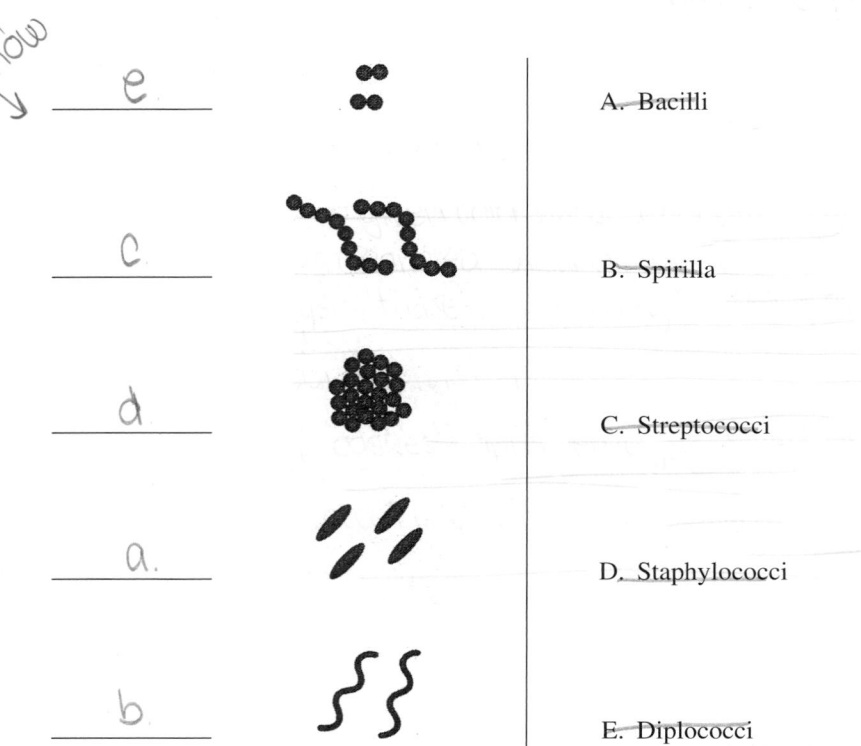

need to know ↓

___e___   A. Bacilli

___c___   B. Spirilla

___d___   C. Streptococci

___a.___   D. Staphylococci

___b___   E. Diplococci

20. Describe the benefits that flagella, spores, and capsules give to organisms that possess these structures.

Flagella allows the organism to be motile.
Spores convert back to a Reproductive stage when conditions improve.
capsules are virulent because antibiotics have difficulty penetrating the capsules.

21. List four ways that a medical assistant can take precautions to prevent the spread of infection to others or to themselves.

wear the appropriate PPE devices. Disinfect specimen containers after collection.
Put the specimens in transport bags after collection. Wash the hands after specimen collection.

22. When is the ideal time to collect a microbiology specimen?

Before antibiotics have been administered because antibiotics will kill the microbes that are needed to be grown and identified.

23. Discuss the Jembec transport system.

It is used for transporting and growing Neisseria gonorrhoeae, the gram-negative diplococcus that causes gonorrhea.

_Cg_

24. Describe the cell wall structures that cause some organisms to be gram positive or gram negative.

_____

_____

25. Give the color of gram-positive and gram-negative organisms after the decolorizer step has been applied.

Gram-positive organisms are purple.

Gram-negative organisms are pink/red.

26. Label the supplies needed for Gram staining (see Procedure 8-2 in the textbook).

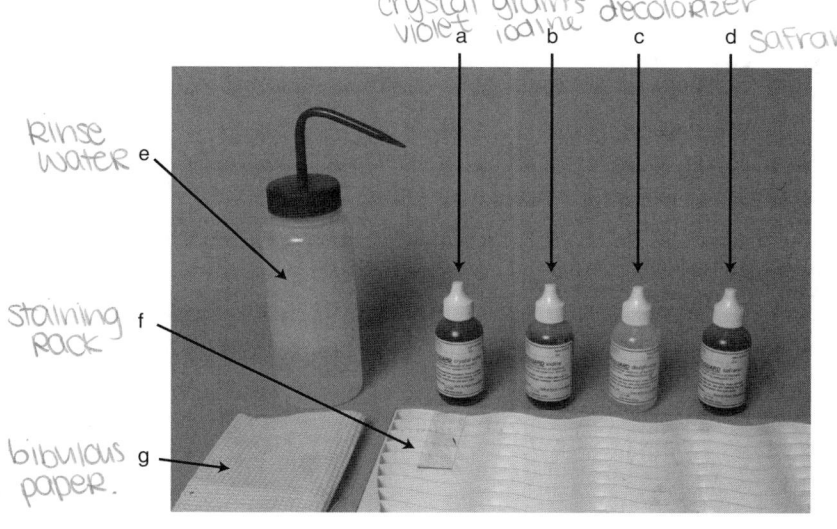

crystal violet a   gram's iodine b   decolorizer c   d safranin

Rinse water e

Staining Rack f

bibulous paper g

27. What is the causative agent for tuberculosis?

Mycobacterium tuberculosis

_____

28. Describe the appearance and characteristics of *Trichomonas vaginalis*.

It's pear-shaped protozoa with 4 flagella that give it a characteristic jerky movement. In women, it causes itching and frothy, creamy discharge in vagina. In men, it's usually asymptomatic and serve as carriers.

29. Case study: On each blank below, write **C** if the statement is correct and **I** if the statement is incorrect. If the step is incorrect, explain why in the space provided.
A medical assistant is performing Gram staining of a specimen.

_____ 1. The specimen is heat fixed to fix the specimen to the slide.

_____

___I___ 2. Crystal violet is applied to the slide for 2 minutes and then rinsed with water.

1 minute.

___C___ 3. Gram's iodine is applied for 1 minute, and both gram-positive and gram-negative organisms are purple. Rinse with water.

_____

_C._ 4. The decolorizer is applied until the purple has stopped running off the slide. This is the most critical step. Rinse with water.

_I._ 5. Safranin is applied last for 1 minute and rinsed with water. Gram-positive organisms are pink or red, and gram-negative organisms are purple.

gram-positive are purple and gram-negative are pink/red.

PROCEDURES: CLINICAL LABORATORY IMPROVEMENT AMENDMENT (CLIA)–WAIVED MICROBIOLOGY TESTS

30. Describe the appearance of alpha, beta, and gamma hemolysis on blood agar plates.

Alpha hemolysis is green color around colonies.
Beta hemolysis is clear area around colonies
Gamma hemolysis there is No hemolysis seen around colonies.

31. State the causative agent (genus and species) of strep throat, and give the most common hemolytic reaction that this organism produces on blood agar plates.

Streptococcus pyogenes. Alpha hemolysis is seen as green color around the colonies.

32. What antibiotic is in the disk that is used to identify *Streptococcus pyogenes*?

Bacitrocin.

33. Label the supplies needed to perform a group A *Streptococcus* test (see Procedure 8-5 in the textbook).

a — Acceava box
b — Reagents 1 + 2
c — positive + negative liquid controls.
d — testing tube
e — test sticks and container
f — sterile swab.

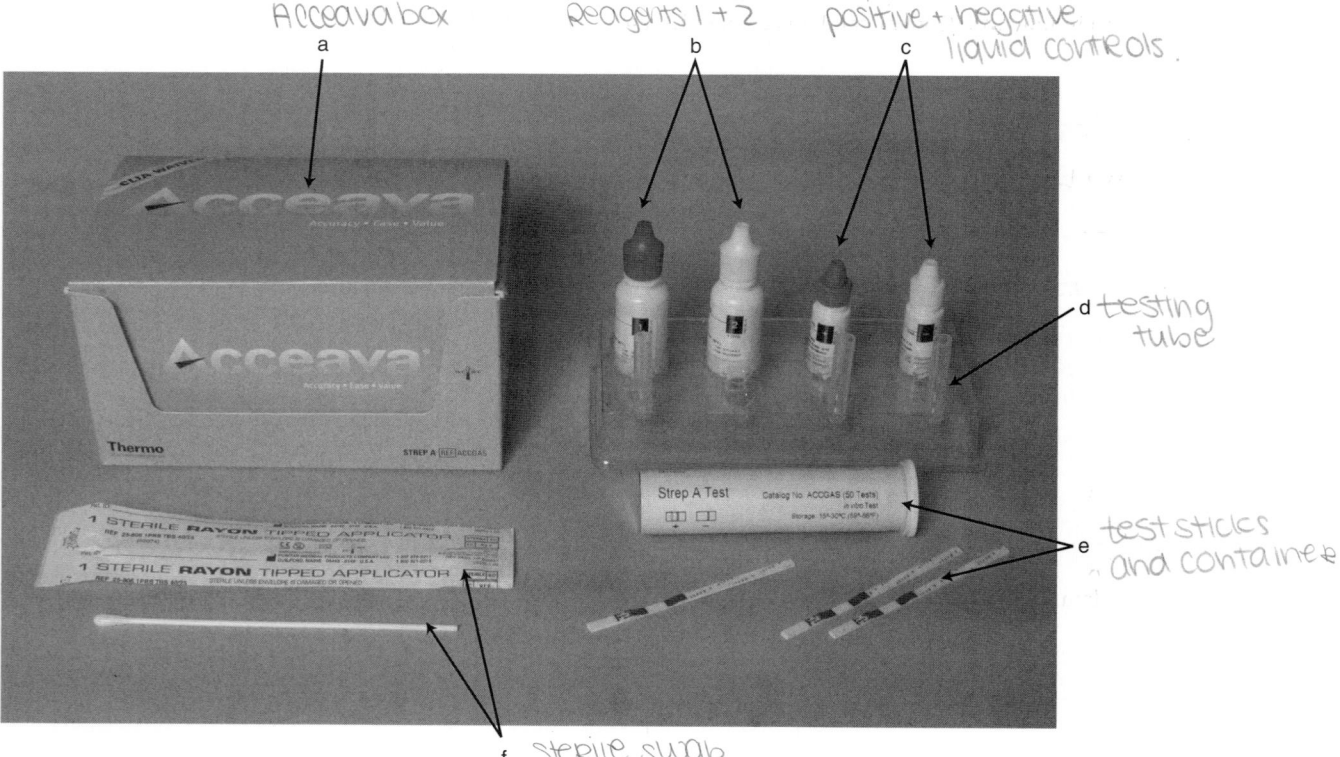

34. List three medical conditions associated with a strep infection.

Scarlet fever, Rheumatic fever, and glomerulonephritis.

35. When discussing influenza, what is the difference between antigenic *drift* and *shift*?

Antigenic drift: gradual change in the virus stain

Antigenic shift: abrupt change in the antigenic properties of the virus.

36. Describe how to obtain a nasal swab specimen when testing for influenza.

A soft foam swab approximately 1 inch into the nose. Swab can then be placed in a dry, closed container for up to 8 hrs.

ADVANCED CONCEPTS

37. Give the oxygen requirements for aerobic, anaerobic, and facultative anaerobic organisms.

Aerobic: require oxygen for growth. Anaerobic: organisms can grow and function in absence of oxygen. Facultative anaerobic: capable of growing in absence of oxygen.

38. Name media requirements that most bacteria need for growth.

Selective media, nutrient media, differential media, and enriched media

39. Explain how MacConkey media is a selective and a differential media.

MacConkey in selective is gram-pos. organisms that are inhibited from growing on this type of media. In differential, it differentiates between bacteria that can ferment the sugar lactose and those that cannot.

40. Describe the shape, arrangement, and Gram stain appearance of *Neisseria gonorrhoeae*.

Chocolate agar containing blood serum, some amino acids, and vitamins.

41. Give the advantages of using an incinerator instead of a Bunsen burner.

It's much safer because it prevents splattering

42. Describe or draw a picture of the differences between quadrant streaking and colony count streaking.

QS: sterilized loop to spread the specimen over 4 areas of plate to establish isolated colonies of bacteria that can be used for id. CCS: Streaking entire plate. It's used for antibiotic testing and consists of using swab that has been dipped in broth

43. Explain a physician's reason for ordering a sensitivity test.

- to determine the type of antibiotics that would be most effective at treating patient's bacterial infections.

containing only one kind of organism and swabbing the entire plate.

165

44. List three organisms that frequently cause urinary tract infections.

Escherichia coli , Proteus spp., Klebsiella spp.

45. Case study: By using Tables 8-3 through 8-9 in the textbook, complete the following information:

Streptococcus pneumoniae
- Gram stain reaction: _gram-positive encapsulated cocci in pairs_
- Disease: _Pneumonia_
- Transmission: _direct contact, droplets._
- Specimens: _sputum, bronchoscopy secretions_

Neisseria gonorrhoeae
- Gram stain reaction: _gram-negative cocci in pairs; intra cellular in WBCs._
- Disease: _Gonorrhea_
- Transmission: _sexual transmitted_
- Specimens: _swab of cervix, urethra rectal and pharyngeal swabs in Homos._

Chlamydia trachomatis
- Disease: _Nongonococcal urethritis and vaginitis_
- Transmission: _sexual_
- Specimens: _swabs for culture and serological testing._

Enterobius vermicularis
- Transmission: _fecal / oral_
- Specimens or tests: _adhesive tape applied to perianal region for ova._

Urinary tract infections
- Organisms: _Eschericha coli, Proteus spp., Klebsiella spp., Pseudomonas aeruginosa._
- Gram stain reaction: _Gram-neg. bacilli, many flagellated_
- Transmission: _ascends urethra; catheterization_
- Tests or specimen: _clean catch urine for culture and analysis_

Food poisoning (most common cause in the United States)
- Organisms: _Campylobacter jejuni_
- Gram stain reaction: _paired gram-neg. curved rods forming a seagull shape_
- Transmission: _contaminated food, water, drink_
- Tests or specimen: _stool for dark field microscopy_

Procedure 8-1: Procedure for Collecting a Throat Specimen

Person evaluated _____   Date _____

Evaluated by _____   Score _____

Outcome goal	To perform throat specimen collection
Conditions	Supplies required: - Sterile swabs and tongue depressor - Personal protective equipment
Standards	Required time = 10 minutes Performance time = _____ Total possible points = _____ Points earned = _____
Evaluation Rubric Codes: **S** = Satisfactory, meets standard **U** = Unsatisfactory, fails to meet standard	
NOTE: Steps marked with an asterisk (*) are critical to achieve required competency.	

Preparation	Scores	
	S	U
*1. Identified patient and placed in proper position.		
- Had patient state name.		
- Confirmed identification with patient.		
- Compared with requisition.		

Procedure	Scores	
	S	U
*2. Sanitized hands and put on gloves and face mask.		
*3. Aseptically removed the sterile Dacron swab (cotton swab may inhibit growth of bacteria) from the package, holding only the tip of the swab.		
4. Had the patient sit with head back.		
*5. Used a sterile tongue depressor to hold down the tongue and had patient say "ahh."		
*6. Rotated the swab on the back of throat in a circular motion or figure-eight pattern.		
- Did not touch the teeth or back of the tongue because these areas have normal flora.		
- Two swabs can be used at the same time: one for a rapid strep test and one for a culture if needed.		
7. Inserted swab into appropriate container for testing.		

Follow-up	Scores	
	S	U
8. Determined if patient was feeling well before dismissing.		
*9. Completed proper documentation on patient chart (see following page).		
*10. Proper disposal and disinfection		

167

- Disinfected test area and instruments according to OSHA guidelines.		
- Disposed regulated medical waste (e.g., gloves, tongue depressor) into biohazard bags.		
*11. Sanitized hands		
Total Points per Column		

Patient Name: _____

Patient Chart Entry: (Include when, what, how, why, any additional information, and the signature of the person charting.)

_____

_____

Procedure 8-2: Gram Stain Procedure

Person evaluated _____   Date _____

Evaluated by _____   Score _____

Outcome goal	Perform a Gram stain
Conditions	Supplies required: - Gloves, bibulous paper, water bottle, or running water - Gram staining reagents: crystal violet, Gram's iodine, decolorizer, safranin - Staining rack
Standards	Required time = 15 minutes Performance time = _____ Total possible points = _____ Points earned = _____ Accuracy = final slide shows gram-positive and gram-negative bacteria

Evaluation Rubric Codes:
S = Satisfactory, meets standard   **U** = Unsatisfactory, fails to meet standard

Preparation	Scores	
	S	**U**
1. Sanitized hands and applied gloves.		
2. Fixed specimen to the slide (using heat or methanol).		

Procedure	Scores	
	S	**U**
3. Applied crystal violet to slide for 1 minute.		
4. Rinsed slide with water.		
5. Applied Gram's iodine to slide for 1 minute.		
6. Rinsed slide with water.		
7. Poured decolorizer over the tilted slide until no more purple ran off (about 3–5 seconds) and then immediately rinsed slide with water to stop the reaction.		
8. Applied safranin stain for 1 minute.		
9. Rinsed slide with water.		
10. Blotted slide dry in absorbent bibulous paper.		

Follow-up	Scores	
	S	**U**
11. Proper disposal and disinfection		
- Disinfected test area and instruments according to OSHA guidelines.		
- Disposed regulated medical waste (e.g., gloves) into biohazard bags.		
- Sanitized hands.		
Total Points per Column		

Chapter **8** **Microbiology**

Procedure 8-5: Acceava Strep A Test Procedure

Person evaluated _____ Date _____

Evaluated by _____ Score _____

Outcome goal	To perform FDA-approved, CLIA-waived rapid strep test following the most current OSHA safety guidelines and applying the correct quality control

Conditions	Supplies required:
	- Acceava rapid strep kit containing:
	  - Reagent 1 and reagent 2
	  - Liquid controls, positive and negative
	  - Soft plastic testing tubes
	  - Test stick and its container
	- Sterile rayon swab taken from wrapper
	- Sterile tongue depressor
	- Gloves, face protection

Standards	Required time = 10 minutes Performance time = _____ Total possible points = _____ Points earned = _____
Evaluation Rubric Codes: **S** = Satisfactory, meets standard **U** = Unsatisfactory, fails to meet standard	
NOTE: Steps marked with an asterisk (*) are critical to achieve required competency.	

Preparation: Preanalytical Phase	Scores	
	S	**U**
A. Test information		
- Kit or instrument method: **Strep A Test**		
- Manufacturer: **Acceava**		
- Proper storage (e.g., temperature, light): **room temperature**		
- Lot # of kit: _____		
- Expiration date: _____		
- Package insert or test flow chart available: _____ yes _____ no		
B. Specimen information		
- Type of specimen: **throat swab using swab from kit (do not use cotton swabs)**		
C. Personal protective equipment: **gloves, facemask during throat swab, and biohazard container**		

Procedure: Analytical Phase	Scores	
	S	**U**
D. Performed/observed qualitative quality control		
- External liquid controls: positive _____ negative _____		
- Internal control: _____ (appears as a red line on test stick)		

	S	U
E. Performed patient test		
1. Sanitized hands and applied gloves.		
2. Just before testing, added three drops of reagent 1 and three drops of reagent 2 into the test tube. The solution should turn light yellow.		
3. Immediately put the throat swab into the extract solution.		
4. Vigorously mixed the solution by rotating the swab forcefully against the side of the tube at least 10 times. Best results are obtained when the specimen is vigorously extracted in the solution.		
5. Let stand for 1 minute, and then squeezed the swab with the sides of the tube as the swab was being withdrawn; discarded the swab into a biohazard container.		
6. Removed a test stick from the container and recapped immediately; placed the absorbent end of the test stick into the extracted sample in the tube.		
7. At 5 minutes, read and recorded the results.		
- Positive = a blue line in test area and pink line in control area, indicating the internal control worked.		
- Negative = no blue line in the test area and a pink line in control area, indicating the internal control worked.		

*Accurate Results _____   Instructor Confirmation _____

Follow-up: Postanalytical Phase	Scores	
	S	U
*F. Proper documentation		
1. On control/patient log: _____ yes _____ no		
2. Documented on patient chart (see below).		
3. Identified critical values and took appropriate steps to notify physician.		
- Expected values for analyte: negative for strep.		
G. Proper disposal and disinfection		
1. Disposed all sharps into biohazard sharps containers.		
2. Disposed all other regulated medical waste into biohazard bags.		
3. Disinfected test area and instruments according to OSHA guidelines.		
4. Sanitized hands after removing gloves.		
Total Points per Column		

Patient Name: _____

Patient Chart Entry: (Include when, what, how, why, any additional information, and the signature of the person charting.)

_____

_____

_____

Procedure 8-6: OSOM Influenza A and B Test Procedure

Person evaluated _____ Date _____

Evaluated by _____ Score _____

Outcome goal	To perform FDA-approved, CLIA-waived influenza test following the most current OSHA safety guidelines and applying the correct quality control
Conditions	Supplies required for the OSOM Influenza A&B Test: - Personal protective equipment (face mask and gloves) - Foam swab provided in kit to collect nasal specimen - Plastic testing tube provided in kit - Extract solution provided in kit - Testing strip provided in kit - Control swabs for influenza A and B - Container of testing strips with diagram showing how to interpret results
Standards	Required time = 10 minutes Performance time = _____ Total possible points = _____ Points earned = _____
Evaluation Rubric Codes: **S** = Satisfactory, meets standard **U** = Unsatisfactory, fails to meet standard	
NOTE: Steps marked with an asterisk (*) are critical to achieve required competency.	

Preparation: Preanalytical Phase	Scores	
	S	U
A. Test information		
- Kit or instrument method: **OSOM A&B Influenza Test**		
- Manufacturer: **Genzyme**		
- Proper storage (e.g., temperature, light): **room temperature**		
- Lot # of kit: _____		
- Expiration date: _____		
- Package insert or test flow chart available: _____ yes _____ no		
B. Specimen information		
- Type of specimen: **nasal swab using swab from kit**		
- **Sanitize hands and apply gloves and facemask**		
- Insert the foam swab provided in the test kit into the patient's nostril displaying the most secretion. Using a gentle rotation, push the swab until resistance is met at the level of the turbinates (at least 1 inch into the nostril). Rotate the swab a few times against the nasal wall and gently rock it back and forth.		
C. Personal protective equipment: **gloves during testing**		

Procedure: Analytical Phase	Scores	
	S	U
D. Performed/observed qualitative quality control		
External swab controls: Positive A _____ Positive B _____		
- Negative A _____ Negative B _____		
- Internal control will appear as a blue line on test stick.		
E. Performed patient test	S	U
1. Sanitized hands and applied gloves.		
2. Placed the nasal swab into the plastic tube containing the designated amount of extraction buffer solution.		
3. Vigorously twisted the swab against the sides and bottom of the tube at least 10 times, which disrupted the virus particles and released the internal viral nucleoproteins into the solution.		
4. Extracted all the solution from the swab by squeezing the plastic tube against the swab while removing it from the tube and disposed of swab properly.		
5. Dipped the influenza test strip into the tube with the extraction buffer, making sure the arrows on the strip were pointing down.		
6. Allowed 10 minutes for migration of the solution across the test area and control area of the strip, which allowed the nucleoproteins from the virus to react with the reagents on the test strip, causing a color reaction.		
7. Read the results for the influenza A and B test.		
- Positive = Result showed a pink or purple line in the A or B test area and a pink line in the internal control area.		
- Negative = Result showed no color change in the A or B test area and a pink line in the internal control area.		
*Accurate Results _____ Instructor Confirmation _____		
Follow-up: Postanalytical Phase	Scores	
	S	U
*F. Proper documentation		
1. On control/patient log: _____ yes _____ no		
2. Documented on patient chart (see following page).		
3. Identified critical values and took appropriate steps to notify physician.		
- Expected values for analyte: negative for influenza A and B		
G. Proper disposal and disinfection		
1. Disposed all sharps into biohazard sharps containers.		
2. Disposed all other regulated medical waste into biohazard bags.		
3. Disinfected test area and instruments according to OSHA guidelines.		
4. Sanitized hands after removing gloves.		
Total Points per Column		

174

Patient name: _____

Patient Chart Entry: (Include when, what, how, why, any additional information, and the signature of the person charting.)

_____

_____

_____

9 Toxicology

VOCABULARY REVIEW

Match each definition with the correct term.

   d   1. idiosyncrasy

   k   2. pharmacokinetics

   a   3. opiates

   f   4. toxicity

   c   5. qualitative drug screening

   i   6. absorption

   e   7. liberation

   g   8. quantitative

   j   9. buprenorphine

   b   10. distribution

   h   11. cannabinoid

   L   12. metabolite

A. Methadone and morphine
B. Blood carrying the drug through the body
C. Measurement that determines if a substance is present or absent
D. Abnormal susceptibility to a drug or other agent that is peculiar to the individual
E. Release of a prescribed drug from its dosage
F. Level at which a drug becomes poisonous in the body
G. Precise measurement of the amount of a substance present in the specimen
H. Marijuana drug screening
I. Passage of a substance through the surface of the body into body fluids and tissues
J. FDA-approved drug for treating opioid drug addiction
K. Movement of drugs through the body from the time of introduction to elimination
L. Substance produced by the metabolism of a drug in the body

FUNDAMENTAL CONCEPTS

13. List three reasons a specimen would be tested in a toxicology laboratory.

    -determine cause of bizarre behavior, unconsciousness, or life threatening.
    -test for drug use in school personnel and students, truck driver, and public
    -test for drug that enhance athletic abillity.

14. List three toxicology responsibilities in the ambulatory care setting.

    Proper collection of blood specimen used
    In office drug screening test
    monitor patient who is on medications

15. Explain three ways an over-the-counter (OTC) drug can become toxic.

    Overdosage, interaction with other drugs, and idiosyncrasy.

16. Define what makes a drug of abuse.

    — illegally obtained

17. When testing for a drug, urine is usually used for a ___*qualitative*___ result, and blood is used for a ___*quantitative*___ result.

18. Describe *chain of custody* when processing a specimen for drug screening.

    person who witnessed the voiding must sign the document, as must every other person who handles the sample

19. Define MRO.

    Medical Review Officer a licensed physician is responsible for recieving lab results and interpreting and evaluating an

20. Explain the results seen on the left side of the urine drug test illustration.

COC ___*negative*___
AMP ___*negative*___
mAMP ___*positive*___

21. Using Table 9-1, write the drug name that matches the following testing codes:

    THC ___*marijuana*___
    COC ___*cocaine*___
    BUP ___*Buprenorphine*___
    OPI ___*Opiates*___
    BAR ___*Barbiturates*___
    BZO ___*Benzodiazepines*___
    MTD ___*Methadone*___
    AMP ___*Amphetamine*___
    OXY ___*Oxycodone*___
    mAMP ___*Methamphetamine*___

22. Why is it important to monitor drug levels during drug therapy?

    To keep it in therapeutic range.

23. From Table 9-4, list the six drug categories that require therapeutic monitoring.

    Antibiotics, anticonvulsants, antidepressants and anti psychotics, antirheumatics, barbiturates, cardiotonics.

24. Place the following pharmokinetic stages in order: metabolism, absorption, liberation, elimination, and distribution

    Liberation, absorption distribution, metabolism, and elimination.

25. Describe drug *half-life*.

    Amount of time necessary to eliminate 50% of a drug.

26. List three environmental poisons that are tested in toxicology.

    Lead posioning, Iron posioning, Chronic exposure to mercury and arsenic posioning.

Procedure 9-1: Assisting with Urine Collection for Drug Screening

Person evaluated _____ Date _____

Evaluated by _____ Score _____

Outcome goal	To assist with urine collection for drug screening
Conditions	Supplies required: - Urine drug screening collection kit with specimen cup with temperature indicator - Urine specimen containers to be sent to the laboratory - Plastic sealable pouch for the two urine specimen containers chain of custody documents - Personal protective equipment
Standards	Required time = 15 minutes Performance time = _____ Total possible points = _____ Points earned = _____

Evaluation Rubric Codes:
S = Satisfactory, meets standard **U** = Unsatisfactory, fails to meet standard

NOTE: Steps marked with an asterisk (*) are critical to achieve required competency.

Preparation	Scores	
	S	U
1. Explain to the patient the purpose of the test and the procedure to be followed for a midstream clean-catch specimen collection.		
- Had patient state name.		
- Obtained a signed consent form from the patient.		
- Compared with requisition.		

Procedure	Scores	
	S	U
2. Sanitized hands and put on gloves and face mask.		
3. A trained professional must witness the voiding of at least 50 mL of urine into the specimen cup provided in the urine collection drug kit.		
4. Originate the chain of custody document at the time of the sample collection. The person who witnessed the voiding must sign the document, as must every other person who handles the sample.		
5. After the collection, verify the temperature of the urine as seen on the indicator at the bottom of the cup, and document it. *Note:* If the temperature of the urine specimen is out of range (too cold), a second specimen must be collected. If the donor refuses to provide the second specimen under direct observation, the collection would be considered a "refusal to test."		
*6. Transfer the specimen to the two containers that must be labeled with the following information: • Full name of the patient • Date and time of collection • Your initials • Initials of the witnessing officer		

	Scores	

7. Place the two sample containers into the sealed plastic pouch, mark it with a notary-style seal or with tamper-proof tape to protect the integrity of the sample, and send the specimen to the toxicology laboratory.		
8. Place the two sample containers into the sealed plastic pouch, mark it with a notary-style seal or with tamper-proof tape to protect the integrity of the sample, and send the specimen to the toxicology laboratory.		
9. If you are trained and qualified to do the testing, proceed with the testing according to laboratory and state regulations.		

Follow-up	Scores	
	S	U
10. After the initial and confirmatory testing is complete, mark the urine sample, reseal it, and securely store it for a minimum of 30 days or for the length of time specified by laboratory protocols.		
11. Completed proper documentation on patient chart (see below).		
12. Proper disposal and disinfection:		
- Disinfected test area and instruments according to OSHA guidelines.		
- Disposed regulated medical waste (e.g., gloves, tongue depressor) into biohazard bags.		
*13. Sanitized hands.		
Total Points per Column		

Patient Name: _____

Patient Chart Entry: (Include when, what, how, why, any additional information, and the signature of the person charting.)

_____

_____

Procedure 9-2: Assisting with Blood Collection for Alcohol Testing

Person evaluated _____   Date _____

Evaluated by _____   Score _____

Outcome goal	To assist with blood collection for alcohol testing
Conditions	Supplies required: - Gray-topped Vacutainer tubes - Venipuncture needle and holder (or syringe and transfer device) - Nonvolatile disinfectant (e.g., benzalkonium [Zephiran], aqueous thimerosal [Merthiolate]) - Gauze - Tourniquet - Gloves - Legally authorized transportation envelope, container, or plastic pouch
Standards	Required time = 15 minutes Performance time = _____ Total possible points = _____ Points earned = _____ Accuracy = final slide shows gram-positive and gram-negative bacteria
Evaluation Rubric Codes: **S** = Satisfactory, meets standard **U** = Unsatisfactory, fails to meet standard	
NOTE: Steps marked with an asterisk (*) are critical to achieve required competency.	

Patient Preparation	Scores	
	S	**U**
1. An officer of the law is present to act as a witness to the procedure.		
2. The patient probably is still under the influence of alcohol, so explain what you will be doing in as concise a manner as possible. *Note:* Do not allow yourself to become irritated by the speech or mannerisms of the patient. Treat the patient with the respect and dignity with which you treat all patients.		

Blood Collection Procedure	Scores	
	S	**U**
Note: The Department of Justice for each state has established uniform standards for the collection, handling, and preservation of blood samples used for alcohol testing. If you are authorized to obtain specimens for forensic analysis, check your laboratory's procedure manual so that you perform the collection *exactly* as required by the uniform standards established for your state.		
3. Sanitize hands, and apply gloves.		
4. Prepare the draw site using Zephiran, aqueous Merthiolate, or another aqueous disinfectant. *Do not use alcohol or other volatile organic disinfectants to clean the skin site.*		
5. Complete the blood draw, filling both tubes with sufficient blood to permit duplicate blood alcohol determinations.		

183

After Collection	Scores	
	S	U
6. Label the two gray-stoppered tubes with the following information: - Full name of the patient - Date and time of collection - Your initials - Initials of the witnessing officer		
7. Give the labeled blood samples to the witnessing officer, who will immediately complete the required information on the transportation envelope, container, or plastic pouch. The officer will then seal it securely. Information on the envelope or container should include the following: - The full name of the patient - Whether the patient is alive or dead - The submitting agency - The geographic location where the blood was drawn (e.g., hospital, clinic, jail) - The name of the person drawing the blood sample - The date and time the blood sample was drawn - The signature of the witnessing officer		
8. After the envelope or container is sealed, it must not be opened, except for analysis. Each person who is subsequently in possession of the sealed sample must sign his or her name in the space provided on the envelope or container (chain of custody). The integrity of the sample must be safeguarded.		
9. Remove gloves, and wash hands.		
Total Points per Column		

Procedure 9-3: Urine Drug Panel Testing Procedure

Person evaluated _____ Date _____

Evaluated by _____ Score _____

Outcome goal	To perform FDA-approved, CLIA-waived drug panel test following the most current OSHA safety guidelines and applying the correct quality control
Conditions	Supplies required: - Gloves - Test card with multiple test strips (five tests are on each side of the card) - Metal pouch containing the test card (check expiration date and temperature)
Standards	Required time = 10 minutes Performance time = _____ Total possible points = _____ Points earned = _____

Evaluation Rubric Codes:
S = Satisfactory, meets standard **U** = Unsatisfactory, fails to meet standard

NOTE: Steps marked with an asterisk (*) are critical to achieve required competency.

Preparation: Preanalytical Phase	Scores	
	S	**U**
A. Test information		
- Kit or instrument method:		
- Manufacturer:		
- Proper storage (e.g., temperature, light): stored the card at 2° to 30° C (check expiration date)		
- Lot # of kit: _____		
- Expiration date: _____		
- Package insert or test flow chart available: _____ yes _____ no		
B. Specimen information		
- Type of specimen: **Fresh urine specimen or specimen that has been stored at 2° to 8° C for up to 48 hours and then brought to room temperature.**		
C. Sanitize the hands, and apply gloves.		
Procedure: Analytical Phase	**S**	**U**
D. Performed/observed qualitative quality control		
- External liquid controls: positive _____ negative _____		
- Internal control: _____ (appears as a red line on test stick)		

E. Performed patient test	S	U
1. Sanitize the hands, and apply gloves.		
2. Remove the test device from its protective pouch, and label it with the patient's identification. *Note*: If the specimen has been stored in the refrigerator, bring it to room temperature before opening to prevent condensation.		
3. Remove the cap from the end of the test card.		
4. With the arrows pointing toward the urine specimen, immerse the strips of the test card vertically into the urine specimen for at least 10 to 15 seconds. **Immerse the strips to at least the level of the wavy lines on the strips but not above the arrows on the test card.**		
5. Place the test card on a nonabsorbent surface, and wait for the colored lines to appear.		
6. At 5 minutes, read and record the results.		
- Positive test result: One distinct pink band appears in the control region (C), with no line in the test region (T).		
- Negative test result: Two pink bands appear, with one pink band in the control region (C) and one pink band in the patient test region (T).		
- Invalid: Pink bands are absent from the control region. Repeat the test with a new device. If the problem persists, call for technical assistance.		
*Accurate Results _____ **Instructor Confirmation** _____		

Follow-up: Postanalytical Phase	Scores	
	S	U
*F. Proper documentation		
1. On control/patient log: _____ yes _____ no		
2. Documented on patient chart (see below).		
3. Identified critical values and took appropriate steps to notify physician.		
- Expected values for analyte: negative for strep		
G. Proper disposal and disinfection		
1. Disposed all sharps into biohazard sharps containers.		
2. Disposed all other regulated medical waste into biohazard bags.		
3. Disinfected test area and instruments according to OSHA guidelines.		
4. Sanitized hands after removing gloves.		
Total Points per Column		

Patient name: _____

Patient Chart Entry: (Include when, what, how, why, any additional information, and the signature of the person charting.)

_____

_____

_____

186

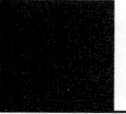

Appendix: Forms for Documenting Safety, Quality Assurance, and CLIA Compliance

CONTENTS

LABORATORY TECH RESPONSIBILITIES

Full Name of Tech	Official Initials	Temp Check Date	Disinfected Counters	Other

188

MONTHLY LABORATORY MAINTENANCE LOG

Medical Clinic							
Daily Maintenance Control Chart							
Month		**Year**					
	Daily				**Monthly**		
Day	**Refrig**	**Freezer**	**Room**	**Incubator**	**Bleach**	**Eye Wash**	**Shower**	**By**
	2-8° C	**0-20° C**	**15-30° C**	**34-36° C**	**Counters**	**Checked**	**Checked**	
1								
2								
3								
4								
5								
6								
7								
8								
9								
10								
11								
12								
13								
14								
15								
16								
17								
18								
19								
20								
21								
22								
23								
24								
25								
26								
27								
28								
29								
30								
31								
Comments								

Exposure Event Number_____

Blood and Body Fluid Exposure Report Form

Facility name: _____

Name of exposed worker: Last: _____ First: _____ ID#: _____

Date of exposure: _____ / _____ / _____   Time of exposure: _____ : _____ AM   PM (Circle)

Job title/occupation: _____ Department/work unit: _____

Location where exposure occurred: _____

Name of person completing form: _____

Section I. Type of Exposure *(Check all that apply.)*

☐ **Percutaneous (Needle or sharp object that was in contact with blood or body fluids)**
   (Complete Sections II, III, IV, and V.)

☐ **Mucocutaneous** *(Check below and complete Sections III, IV, and VI.)*
   ___ **Mucous Membrane**   ___ **Skin**

☐ **Bite** *(Complete Sections III, IV, and VI.)*

Section II. Needle/Sharp Device Information

   (If exposure was percutaneous, provide the following information about the device involved.)

Name of device: _____   ☐ Unknown/Unable to determine

Brand/manufacturer: _____   ☐ Unknown/Unable to determine

Did the device have a sharps injury prevention feature, i.e., a "safety device"?

☐ Yes   ☐ No   ☐ Unknown/Unable to determine

If yes, when did the injury occur?

☐ Before activation of safety feature was appropriate   ☐ Safety feature failed after activation

☐ During activation of the safety feature   ☐ Safety feature not activated

☐ Safety feature improperly activated   ☐ Other:_____

Describe what happened with the safety feature, e.g., why it failed or why it was not activated: _____

_____

Section III. Employee Narrative *(Optional)*

Describe how the exposure occurred and how it might have been prevented:

_____

_____

_____

NOTE: This is not a CDC or OSHA form. This form was developed by CDC to help healthcare facilities with detailed exposure information that is specifically useful for the facilities' prevention planning. Information on this page (#1) may meet OSHA sharps injury documentation requirements and can be copied and filed for purposes of maintaining a separate sharps injury log. Procedures for maintaining employee confidentiality must be followed.

(Courtesy of Centers for Disease Control and Prevention,
http://www.cdc.gov/sharpssafety/pdf/AppendixA-7.doc)

Exposure Event Number_____

Section IV. Exposure and Source Information

A.   **Exposure Details:** *(Check all that apply.)*

1. **Type of fluid or material (For body fluid exposures <u>only</u>, check which fluid in adjacent box.)**

   ☐ Blood/blood products

   ☐ Visibly bloody body fluid*

   ☐ Non-visibly bloody body fluid*

   ☐ Visibly bloody solution (e.g., water used to clean a blood spill)

*Identify which body fluid		
___ Cerebrospinal	___ Urine	___ Synovial
___ Amniotic	___ Sputum	___ Peritoneal
___ Pericardial	___ Saliva	___ Semen/Vaginal
___ Pleural	___ Feces/stool	___ Other/Unknown

2. **Body site of exposure.** *(Check all that apply.)*

   ☐ Hand/finger   ☐ Eye   ☐ Mouth/nose   ☐ Face

   ☐ Arm   ☐ Leg   ☐ Other (Describe:_____)

3. **If percutaneous exposure:**

   Depth of injury *(Check only one.)*

   ☐ Superficial (e.g., scratch, no or little blood)

   ☐ Moderate (e.g., penetrated through skin, wound bled)

   ☐ Deep (e.g., intramuscular penetration)

   ☐ Unsure/Unknown

   Was blood visible on device before exposure?   ☐ Yes   ☐ No   ☐ Unsure/Unknown

4. **If mucous membrane or skin exposure:** *(Check only one.)*

   Approximate volume of material

   ☐ Small (e.g., few drops)

   ☐ Large (e.g., major blood splash)

   If skin exposure, was skin intact?   ☐ Yes   ☐ No   ☐ Unsure/Unknown

B.   **Source Information**

1. **Was the source individual identified?**   ☐ Yes   ☐ No   ☐ Unsure/Unknown

2. **Provide the serostatus of the source patient for the following pathogens.**

	Positive	Negative	Refused	Unknown
HIV Antibody	☐	☐	☐	☐
HCV Antibody	☐	☐	☐	☐
HbsAg	☐	☐	☐	☐

3. **If known, when was the serostatus of the source determined?**

   ☐ Known at the time of exposure

   ☐ Determined through testing at the time of or soon after the exposure

Appendix: Forms for Documenting Safety, Quality Assurance

Exposure Event Number_____

Section V. Percutaneous Injury Circumstances

A. **What device or item caused the injury?**

Hollow-bore needle

☐ Hypodermic needle

__ Attached to syringe __ Attached to IV tubing
__ Unattached

☐ Prefilled cartridge syringe needle

☐ Winged steel needle (i.e., butterfly type devices)

__ Attached to syringe, tube holder, or IV tubing
__ Unattached

☐ IV stylet

☐ Phlebotomy needle

☐ Spinal or epidural needle

☐ Bone marrow needle

☐ Biopsy needle

☐ Huber needle

☐ Other type of hollow-bore needle (type: _____)

☐ Hollow-bore needle, type unknown

Suture needle

☐ Suture needle

Glass

☐ Capillary tube

☐ Pipette (glass)

☐ Slide

☐ Specimen/test/vacuum

☐ Other: _____

Other sharp objects

☐ Bone chip/chipped tooth

☐ Bone cutter

☐ Bovie electrocautery device

☐ Bur

☐ Explorer

☐ Extraction forceps

☐ Elevator

☐ Histology cutting blade

☐ Lancet

☐ Pin

☐ Razor

☐ Retractor

☐ Rod (orthopaedic applications)

☐ Root canal file

☐ Scaler/curette

☐ Scalpel blade

☐ Scissors

☐ Tenaculum

☐ Trocar

☐ Wire

☐ Other type of sharp object

☐ Sharp object, type unknown

Other device or item

☐ Other: _____

B. **Purpose or procedure for which sharp item was used or intended.**
(Check one procedure type and complete information in corresponding box as applicable.)

☐ Establish intravenous or arterial access (Indicate type of line.)——————▶

☐ Access established intravenous or arterial line
(Indicate type of line and reason for line access.)——————▶

☐ Injection through skin or mucous membrane
(Indicate type of injection.) ——————▶

☐ Obtain blood specimen (through skin)
(Indicate method of specimen collection.)——————▶

☐ Other specimen collection

☐ Suturing

☐ Cutting

☐ Other procedure

☐ Unknown

Type of Line	
__ Peripheral	__ Arterial
__ Central	__ Other

Reason for Access
__ Connect IV infusion/piggyback
__ Flush with heparin/saline
__ Obtain blood specimen
__ Inject medication
__ Other: _____

Type of Injection	
__ IM Injection	__ Epidural/spinal anesthesia
__ Skin test placement	__ Other injection
__ Other ID/SQ injection	

Type of Blood Sampling	
__ Venipuncture	__ Umbilical vessel
__ Arterial puncture	__ Finger/heelstick
__ Dialysis/AV fistula site	__ Other blood sampling

192

Exposure Event Number_____

C. **When and how did the injury occur? (From the left hand side of page, select the point during or after use that most closely represents when the injury occurred. In the corresponding right hand box, select *one* or *two* circumstances that reflect how the injury happened.)**

☐ During use of the item ⟶

Select one or two choices:

— Patient moved and jarred device
— While inserting needle/sharp
— While manipulating needle/sharp
— While withdrawing needle/sharp
— Passing or receiving equipment
— Suturing
— Tying sutures
— Manipulating suture needle in holder
— Incising
— Palpating/exploring
— Collided with co-worker or other during procedure
— Collided with sharp during procedure
— Sharp object dropped during procedure

☐ After use, before disposal of item ⟶

Select one or two choices:

— Handling equipment on a tray or stand
— Transferring specimen into specimen container
— Processing specimens
— Passing or transferring equipment
— Recapping (missed or pierced cap)
— Cap fell off after recapping
— Disassembling device or equipment
— Decontamination/processing of used equipment
— During clean-up
— In transit to disposal
— Opening/breaking glass containers
— Collided with co-worker/other person
— Collided with sharp after procedure
— Sharp object dropped after procedure
— Struck by detached IV line needle

☐ During or after disposal of item ⟶

Select one or two choices:

— Placing sharp in container:
  — Injured by sharp being disposed
  — Injured by sharp already in container
— While manipulating container
— Over-filled sharps container
— Punctured sharps container
— Sharp protruding from open container
— Sharp in unusual location:
  — In trash
  — In linen/laundry
  — Left on table/tray
  — Left in bed/mattress
  — On floor
  — In pocket/clothing
  — Other unusual location
— Collided with co-worker or other person
— Collided with sharp
— Sharp object dropped
— Struck by detached IV line needle

☐ Other (Describe): _____

_____

_____

_____

☐ Unknown

193

Exposure Event Number_____

Section VI.   Mucous Membrane Exposures Circumstances

A.   **What barriers were used by worker at the time of the exposure?** *(Check all that apply.)*

☐ Gloves   ☐ Goggles   ☐ Eyeglasses   ☐ Face Shield   ☐ Mask   ☐ Gown

B.   **Activity/Event when exposure occurred** *(Check one.)*

☐ Patient spit/coughed/vomited
☐ Airway manipulation (e.g., suctioning airway, inducing sputum)
☐ Endoscopic procedure
☐ Dental procedure
☐ Tube placement/removal/manipulation (e.g., chest, endotracheal, NG, rectal, urine catheter)
☐ Phlebotomy
☐ IV or arterial line insertion/removal/manipulation
☐ Irrigation procedure
☐ Vaginal delivery
☐ Surgical procedure (e.g., all surgical procedures including C-section)
☐ Bleeding vessel
☐ Changing dressing/wound care
☐ Manipulating blood tube/bottle/specimen container
☐ Cleaning/transporting contaminated equipment
☐ Other: _____
☐ Unknown

Comments: _____

_____

_____

_____

_____

_____

_____

_____

GENERIC QUALITATIVE CONTROL AND PATIENT LOG (TEMPLATE)

Test: _____

Kit Name and Manufacturer: _____

Lot #: _____   Expiration Date: _____

Storage Requirements: _____   Test Flow Chart: _____

Date	Specimen ID (Control/Patient)	Result (+ or −)	Internal Control Passed (Y or N)	Charted in Patient Record	Tech Initials

Appendix: Forms for Documenting Safety, Quality Assurance

GENERIC QUANTITATIVE TEST CONTROL LOG (TEMPLATE)

Control Lot #: _____   Expiration Date _____

Control Range: _____   Control Level: _____

Date	Tech	Result	Accept	Reject	Corrective Action

MONTHLY LEVY-JENNINGS QC CHART

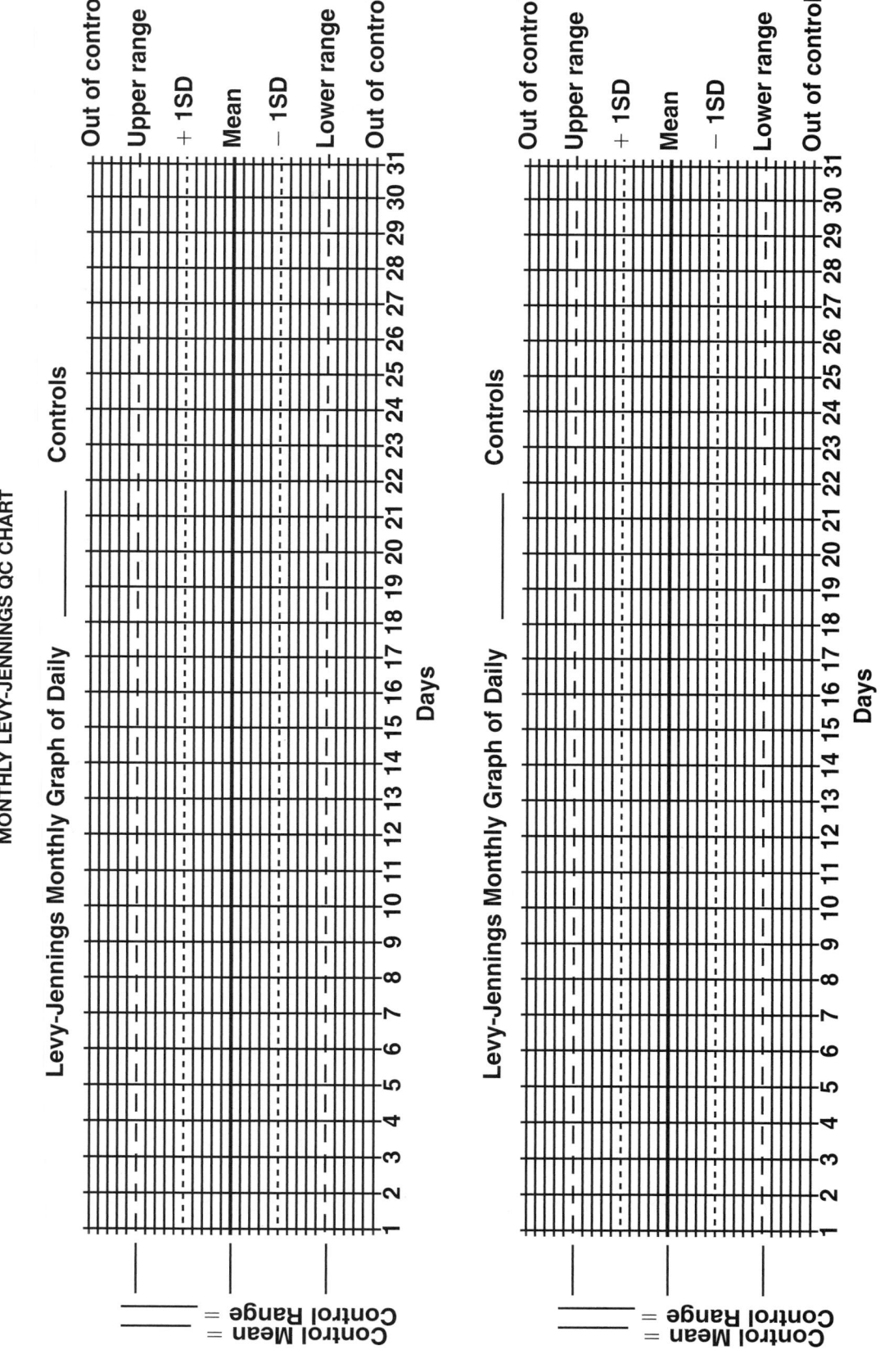

Levy-Jennings Monthly Graph of Daily _____ Controls

Days

Control Mean = _____
Control Range = _____

Out of control
Upper range
+ 1SD
Mean
– 1SD
Lower range
Out of control

Levy-Jennings Monthly Graph of Daily _____ Controls

Days

Control Mean = _____
Control Range = _____

Out of control
Upper range
+ 1SD
Mean
– 1SD
Lower range
Out of control

URINE DIPSTICK QUALITY CONTROL LOG

DATE _____ URINE DIPSTICK CONTROL LEVEL _____ LOT # _____ EXPIRATION DATE _____

DATE	Reagent Strip Lot # Patient	DIPSTICK TESTS											CONFIRMATORY TESTS								ADD. TESTS		INITIAL
		Leukocytes	Nitrites	Urobilinogen	Protein	pH	Blood	Specific Gravity	Ketones	Bilirubin	Glucose	Protein	Method/Lot #	Ketones	Method/Lot #	Glucose	Method/Lot #	Bilirubin	Method/Lot #	hCG	Method/Lot #	Specific Gravity Refractometer	

(From Zakus SM: *Clinical skills for medical assistants*, ed 4, St. Louis, 2001, Mosby.)

URINE DIPSTICK PATIENT LOG

DATE	Reagent Strip / Lot# / Patient	DIPSTICK TESTS											CONFIRMATORY TESTS								ADD. TESTS		INITIAL
		Leukocytes	Nitrites	Urobilinogen	Protein	pH	Blood	Specific Gravity	Ketones	Bilirubin	Glucose	Protein	Method/Lot #	Ketones	Method/Lot #	Glucose	Method/Lot #	Bilirubin	Method/Lot #	hCG	Method/Lot #	Specific Gravity Refractometer	

(From Zakus SM: *Clinical skills for medical assistants*, ed 4, St. Louis, 2001, Mosby.)

Appendix: Forms for Documenting Safety, Quality Assurance

Sample Device Pre-Selection Worksheet

Type of Device: _____   **Name:** _____   **Manufacturer:** _____

Clinical Considerations		Does this consideration apply to this device?		If Yes, what is the level of importance?		
		No	Yes	High	Med	Low
Procedural Implications for Healthcare Provider	Device use will require a change in technique (compared to conventional product).					
	Device permits needle changes.					
	Device permits reuse of the needle on the same patient during a procedure. (e.g., local anesthesia)					
	Device allows easy visualization of flashback.					
	Device allows easy visualization of medication.					
	Other:					
	Comment:					

Clinical Considerations		Does this consideration apply to this device?		If Yes, what is the level of importance?		
		No	Yes	High	Med	Low
Patient Considerations	Device is latex free.					
	Device has potential for causing infection.					
	Device has potential for causing increased pain or discomfort to patients.					
	Other:					
	Comment:					
Scope of Device Use Considerations	Device can be used with adult and pediatric populations.					
	Specialty areas (e.g., OR, anesthesiology, radiology) can use the device.					
	Device can be used for all same purposes for which the conventional device is used.					
	Device is available in all currently used sizes.					
	Other:					
	Comment:					

Safety Considerations	Does this consideration apply to this device?		If Yes, what is the level of importance?		
	No	Yes	High	Med	Low
Method Activation					
The safety feature does not require activation by the user.					
The worker's hands can remain behind the sharp during activation of the safety.					
Activation of the safety feature can be performed with one hand.					
Other:					
Comment:					
Characteristics of the Safety Feature					
The safety feature is in effect during use in the patient.					
The safety feature permanently isolates the sharp.					
The safety feature is integrated into the device (i.e., does not need to be added before use).					
A visible or audible cue provides evidence of safety feature activation.					
The safety feature is easy to recognize and intuitive to use.					
Other:					
Comment:					

Other Considerations		Does this consideration apply to this device?		If Yes, what is the level of importance?		
		No	Yes	High	Med	Low
Availability	The device is available in all sizes currently used in the organization.					
	The manufacturer can provide the device in needed quantities.					
Service Provided	The company representative will assist with training.					
	Product materials are available to assist with training.					
	The company will provide free samples for evaluation.					
	The company has a history of being responsive when problems arise.					
	Comment:					
Practical Considerations	The device will **not** increase the volume of sharps waste.					
	The device will **not** require changes in the size or shape of sharps containers.					
	Other:					
	Comment:					

Courtesy of Centers for Disease Control and Prevention, "Sample Device Pre-Selection Worksheet," Sharps Injury Prevention Workbook, A-12, http://www.cdc.gov/sharpssafety/index.html.

Appendix: Forms for Documenting Safety, Quality Assurance

SAMPLE DEVICE EVALUATION FORM

Product: _____   Date: _____

Department/unit: _____   Position/title: _____

1. **Number of times you used the device.**

   ☐ 1–5   ☐ 6–10   ☐ 11–25   ☐ 26–50   ☐ More than 50

2. Please mark the box that best describes your experiences with the device. If a question is not applicable to this device, do not fill in an answer for that question.

Factors	Strongly Disagree	Disagree	Neither Agree nor Disagree	Agree	Strongly Agree
Patient/Procedure Considerations					
a. Needle penetration **is** comparable to the standard device.	1	2	3	4	5
b. Patients/residents **do not** perceive more pain or discomfort with this device.	1	2	3	4	5
c. Use of the device **does not** increase the number of repeat sticks of patient.	1	2	3	4	5
d. The device **does not** increase the time it takes to perform the procedure.	1	2	3	4	5
e. Use of the device **does not** require a change in procedural technique.	1	2	3	4	5
f. The device is compatible with other equipment that must be used with it.	1	2	3	4	5
g. The device can be used for the same purposes as the standard device.	1	2	3	4	5
h. Use of the device **is not** affected by my hand size.	1	2	3	4	5
i. Age or size of patient/resident **does not** affect use of this device.	1	2	3	4	5
Experience with the Safety Feature					
j. Safety feature **does not** interfere with procedural technique.	1	2	3	4	5
k. The safety feature is easy to activate.	1	2	3	4	5
l. Safety feature **does not** activate before the procedure is completed.	1	2	3	4	5
m. Once activated, the safety feature remains engaged.	1	2	3	4	5
n. I **did not** experience any injury or *near miss* of injury with the device.	1	2	3	4	5
Special Questions about this Particular Device					

[To be added by health care facility]	1	2	3	4	5
	1	2	3	4	5
	1	2	3	4	5
Overall Rating					
Overall, the device is effective for both patient/resident care and safety.	1	2	3	4	5

3. Did you participate in training on how to use this product?

☐ No *(Go to question 6.)*   ☐ Yes *(Go to next question.)*

4. Who provided this instruction? *(Check all that apply.)*

☐ Product representative   ☐ Staff development personnel   ☐ Other _____

5. Was the training you received adequate?

☐ No   ☐ Yes

6. Was special training needed to use the product effectively?

☐ No   ☐ Yes

7. Compared with others of your gender, how would you describe your hand size?

☐ Small   ☐ Medium   ☐ Large

8. What is your gender?

☐ Female   ☐ Male

9. Which of the following do you consider yourself to be?

☐ Left-handed   ☐ Right-handed

10. Please add any additional comments below.

_____

_____

THANK YOU FOR COMPLETING THIS SURVEY

Please return this form to:_____

(Courtesy of Centers for Disease Control and Prevention, Sample Device Evaluation Form, Sharps Injury Prevention Workbook, A-13; http://www.cdc.gov/sharpssafety/index.html)

Quality Control Flow Chart for HemoCue

Regardless of the purpose, most clinical testing procedures have the same quality control requirements. If an instrument is used, there is usually a method to check its mechanical function. Often this is nothing more than an "optic check" or calibration strip supplied with the instrument to allow the user to determine whether the instrument is functional.

After determining that the instrument does indeed function, one then needs to prove that the reagents will perform as expected. Commonly, one uses a high and low value control sample. Look at the results. Are they within their expected ranges? If so, you can begin to test patients. If not, then it is time to do some troubleshooting.

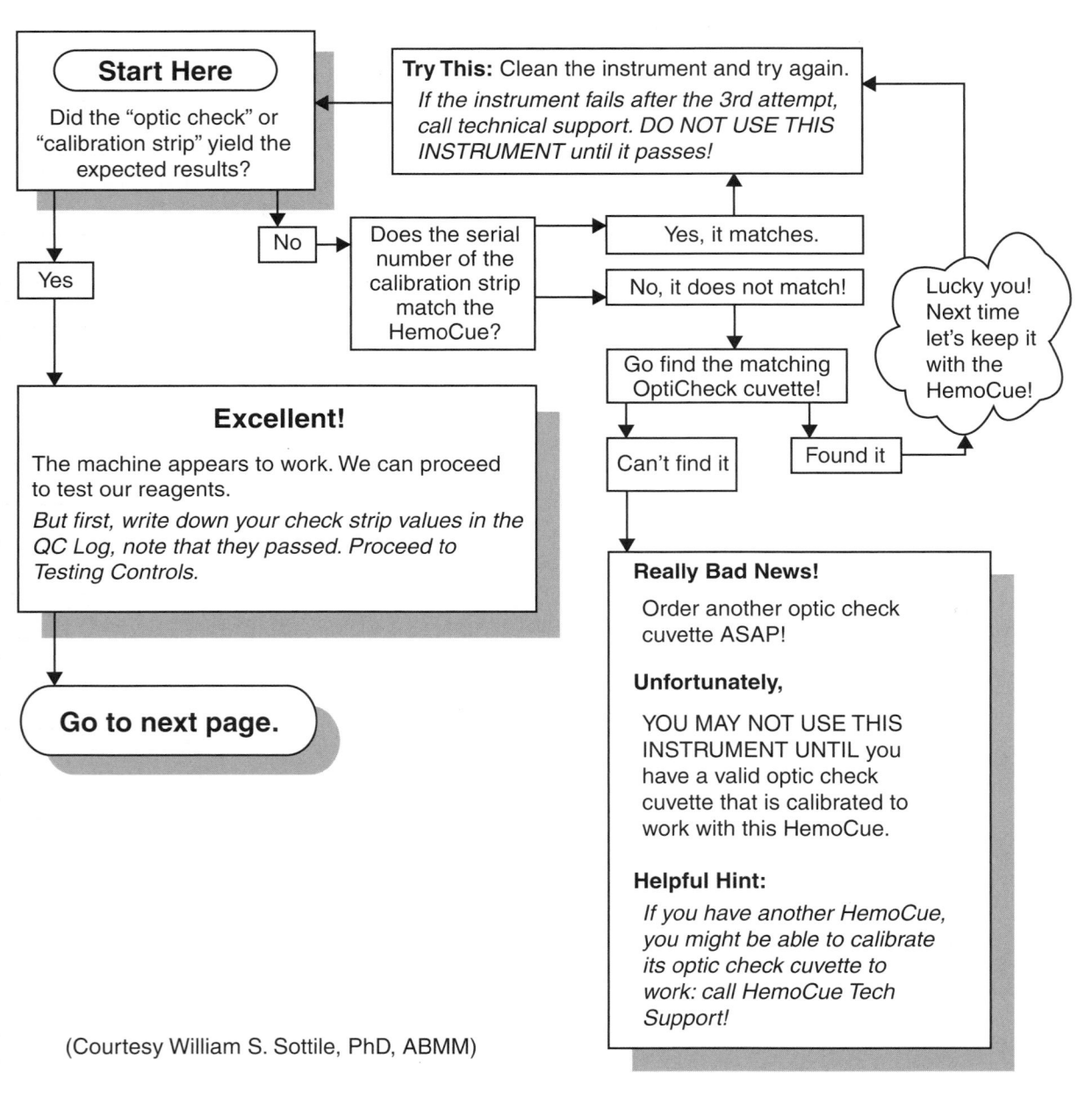

(Courtesy William S. Sottile, PhD, ABMM)

HEMOGLOBIN QUALITY CONTROL LOG

Test: _____ Control Lot #: _____

Control Range: _____ For Low/Normal/High Control

Date	Tech	Result	Accept	Reject	Corrective Action

HEMOGLOBIN PATIENT LOG

Test: _____   Kit Lot #: _____

Expected Hemoglobin Values:

Adult males = 13.0–18 g/dL   Adult females = 11.0–16.0 g/dL

Infants = 10.0–14.0 g/dL   Children = Increase to adult

Date	Tech	Patient ID	Result	Charted

HEMATOCRIT QUALITY CONTROL LOG

Test: _____

Control Range : _____

Control Lot #: _____

For Low/Normal/High Control

Date	Tech	Slot #	Result	Accept	Reject	Corrective Action

Appendix: Forms for Documenting Safety, Quality Assurance

HEMATOCRIT PATIENT LOG

Expected Hematocrit Values:

Adult males = 42–52%   Adult females = 36–48%

Infants = 32–38%   Children = Increase to adult

Date	Tech	Patient ID	Slot #	Result	Charted

ERYTHROCYTE SEDIMENTATION RATE PATIENT LOG

Expected ESR Values:

Adult males < 50 yr = 0–15 mm/hr   Adult females < 50 yr = 0–20 mm/hr

Adult males > 50 yr = 0–20 mm/hr   Adult females > 50 yr = 0–30 mm/hr

Date	Tech	Patient ID	Slot #	Time	Result	Charted

Appendix: Forms for Documenting Safety, Quality Assurance

PROTIME PATIENT LOG

ProTime expected values for normal and therapeutic whole blood:

	INR	PT (seconds; see ranges in insert)
Normal	0.8–1.2	_____
Low anticoagulation	1.5–2.0	_____
Moderate anticoagulation	2.0–3.0	_____
High anticoagulation	2.5–4.0	_____

Date	Tech	Patient ID	INR	PT (seconds)	Charted

GLUCOSE TEST CONTROL LOG

Control Lot #: _____   Expiration Date: _____

Control Range: _____   Level: Low/Normal/High

Date	Tech	Result	Accept	Reject	Corrective Action

Appendix: Forms for Documenting Safety, Quality Assurance

GLUCOSE PATIENT LOG

Date	Patient	Result	Charted	Tech

HEMOGLOBIN A1c PATIENT/CONTROL LOG

Date	Patient	Result	Charted	Tech

Appendix: Forms for Documenting Safety, Quality Assurance

CHOLESTECH LDX PATIENT/CONTROL LOG

Cassette Lot #: _____   **Expiration Date:** _____   **LDX Serial #:** _____

Date	Operator	Patient ID	Charted	TRG	TC	GLU	HDL	LDL	TC/HDL	ALT

HEMOCCULT PATIENT LOG

Date	Patient	Result	Tech

Appendix: Forms for Documenting Safety, Quality Assurance

I-STAT PATIENT/CONTROL LOG

Cartridge Lot #:_____   Expiration Date: _____   Serial #: _____

Date	Operator	Patient ID	Charted	Na	K	Cl	TCO$_2$	iCa	Glu	BUN	Crea	Hct	Hb	AnGap

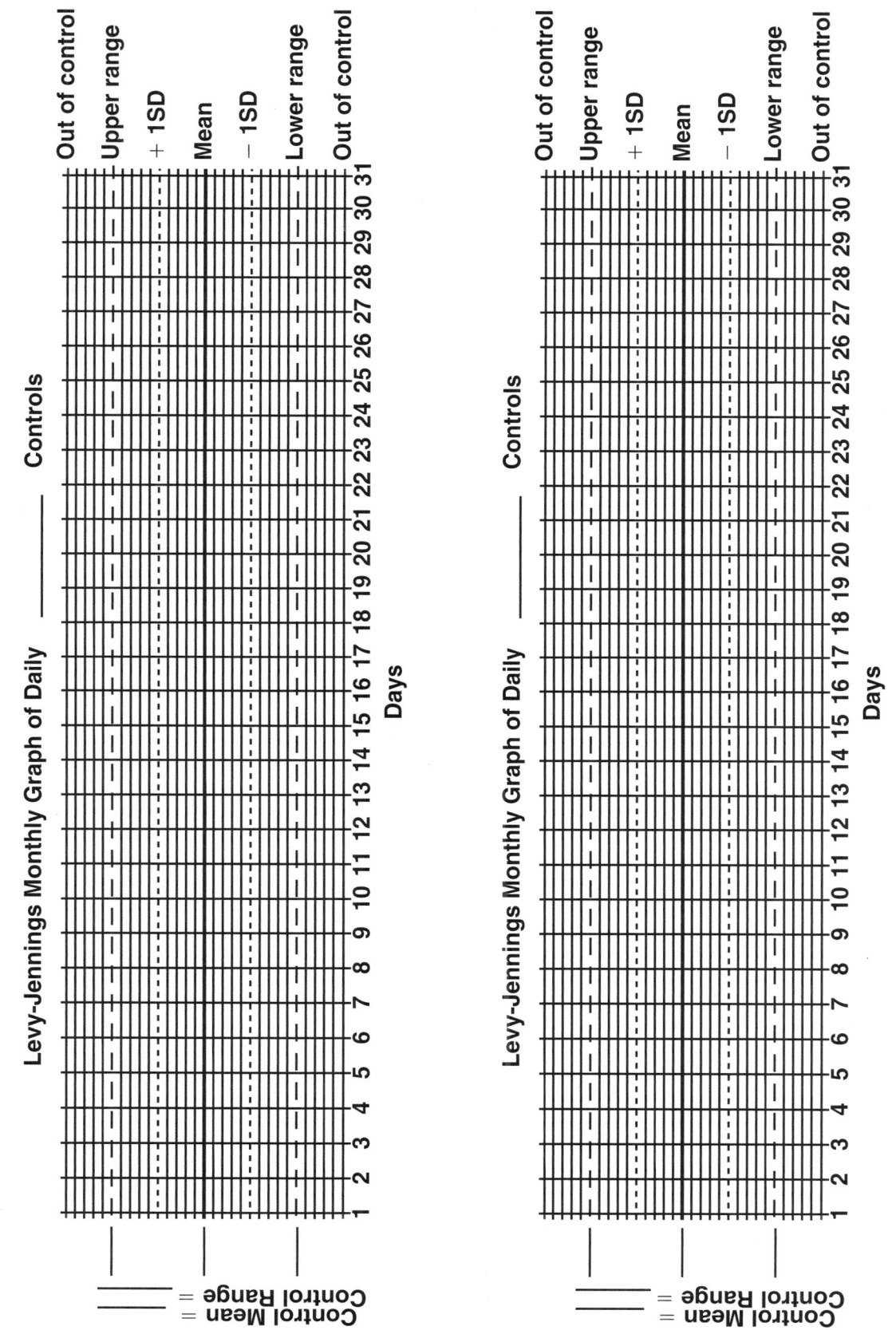

Appendix: Forms for Documenting Safety, Quality Assurance

QUALITATIVE CONTROL AND PATIENT LOG FOR IMMUNOLOGY AND MICROBIOLOGY TEST KITS (TEMPLATE)

Test: _____

Kit Name and Manufacturer: _____

Lot # _____   Expiration Date: _____

Storage Requirements: _____   Test Flow Chart: _____

Date	Specimen ID (Control/Patient)	Result (+ or −)	Internal Control Passed (Y or N)	Charted in Patient Record	Tech Initials

GENERIC QUALITATIVE TEST PROCEDURE (TEMPLATE)

Qualitative Test _____

Person evaluated _____ **Date** _____

Evaluated by _____ **Score** _____

Outcome goal:	Supplies required:	
Conditions:	Required time = _____ minutes	Performance time = _____
Standards:	Total possible points = _____	Points earned = _____

Evaluation Rubric Codes:
S = Satisfactory - Meets standard   **U** = Unsatisfactory - Fails to meet standard

NOTE: Steps marked with an asterisk (*) are critical to achieve required competency.

Preparation: Preanalytical Phase	Scores	
	S	**U**
A. Test information		
- Kit method:		
- Manufacturer:		
- Proper storage (e.g., temperature, light):		
- Lot number of kit: _____		
- Expiration date: _____		
- Package insert and/or test flow chart available: _____ yes _____ no		
B. Personal protective equipment		
C. Specimen information		

Procedure: Analytical Phase	Scores	
	S	**U**
D. Performed/observed qualitative quality control		
- External liquid controls: Positive _____ Negative _____		
- Internal control:		
E. Performed patient test	**S**	**U**
1.		
2.		
3.		
4.		

Appendix: Forms for Documenting Safety, Quality Assurance

	Scores	
POSITIVE seen as:		
NEGATIVE seen as:		
INVALID seen as:		
*Accurate Results _____ Instructor Confirmation _____		
Follow-up: Postanalytical Phase	**S**	**U**
*F. Proper documentation		
1. On control/patient log: _____ yes _____ no		
2. Documentation on patient chart (see below).		
3. Identified "critical values" and took appropriate steps to notify physician EXPECTED VALUES FOR ANALYTE: NEGATIVE		
G. Proper disposal and disinfection		
1. Disposed all sharps into biohazard sharps containers.		
2. Disposed all other regulated medical waste into biohazard bags.		
3. Disinfected test area and instruments according to OSHA guidelines.		
4. Sanitized hands after removing gloves.		
Total Points per Column		

Patient Name: _____

Patient Chart Entry: (Include when, what, how, why, any additional information, and the signature of the person charting.)

_____

_____

_____

GENERIC QUANTITATIVE TEST PROCEDURE (TEMPLATE)

Qualitative Test _____

Person evaluated _____ **Date** _____

Evaluated by _____ **Score** _____

Outcome goal:	
Conditions:	
Standards:	Required time = _____ minutes Performance time = _____ Total possible points = _____ Points earned = _____

Evaluation Rubric Codes:
S = Satisfactory - Meets standard   **U** = Unsatisfactory - Fails to meet standard

NOTE: Steps marked with an asterisk (*) are critical to achieve required competency.

Preparation: Preanalytical Phase	Scores	
	S	**U**
A. Test information		
- Kit or instrumental method: _____		
- Manufacturer: _____		
- Proper storage (e.g., temperature, light): _____		
- Lot number of kit or supplies: _____		
- Expiration date: _____		
- Package insert and/or test flow chart available: _____ yes no _____		
B. Specimen information		
- Type of specimen and its preparation (e.g., fasting, first morning): _____		
- Specimen container or testing device: _____		
- Amount of specimen: _____		
C. Personal protective equipment (PPE): _____		
D. Assembled all the above, sanitized hands, and applied PPE		
Procedure: Analytical Phase	**Scores**	
	S	**U**
E. Performed/observed quality control		
Quantitative testing controls		
- Calibration check: _____		
- Control levels: Normal _____ High _____ Low _____		

223

F. Performed patient test: Followed proper steps (see flow chart and list steps)	S	U
1.		
2.		
3.		
4.		
5.		
6.		
7.		
8.		
9.		
10.		

*Accurate Results _____   Instructor Confirmation _____

Follow-up: Postanalytical	Scores	
	S	U
*G. Proper documentation		
1. On control log _____ yes _____ no		
2. On patient log _____ yes _____ no		
3. Documentation on patient chart (see below)		
4. Identified "critical values" and took appropriate steps to notify physician		
EXPECTED VALUES FOR ANALYTE:		
H. Proper disposal and disinfection		
1. Disposed all sharps into biohazard sharps containers		
2. Disposed all other regulated medical waste into biohazard bags		
3. Disinfected test area and instruments according to OSHA guidelines		
4. Sanitized hands after removing gloves		
Column Totals		

Patient Chart Entry: (Include when, what, how, why, any additional information, and the signature of the person charting.)

_____

_____

_____

PROFESSIONAL EVALUATION FORM FOR THE LABORATORY CLASSROOM

Student: _____ **Date:** _____

Class: _____ **Semester:** _____

Number of Tardies: _____ **Number of Hours Absent:** _____

Objective	Very Satisfactory 3	Satisfactory 2	Unsatisfactory 1	Comments
Exhibits professional written communication (e.g., appearance, language, grammar).				
Uses the class materials appropriately (e.g., equipment, supplies, computers, cleanup).				
Provides instructor with all necessary information in a timely and organized manner (e.g., meets due dates, make-ups turned in within a week).				
Adheres to specific course policies (e.g., make-up guidelines, skill check-offs, externship guidelines).				
Projects a positive attitude and motivation (e.g., seen during lectures and labs).				
Displays professional verbal communication at all times (e.g., respectful, tactful).				
Maintains confidentiality of all personal interactions at all times (see rules of confidentiality in handbook).				
Projects professional work ethics (e.g., responsible, accountable, independent, full use of lab time: practice, study, computer).				
Cooperates with fellow students (e.g., team projects, skill practice, study groups).				
Displays responsible attendance behavior (e.g., arriving on time, calling in if detained or absent, prepared for next class session).				
Dresses appropriately (see handbook).				

Additional Comments:

_____

_____

_____

Student Signature _____ **Instructor** _____

Appendix: Forms for Documenting Safety, Quality Assurance

SAMPLE HEALTH ASSESSMENT FORM

Please print clearly: Date _____

Name _____   Address _____

City _____   State _____   ZIP _____

Telephone _____   Age (date of birth) ____/ ____/ ____

Sex _____   Race _____   Ht. _____   Wt._____

Do you consider yourself overweight? _____   If so, how much? _____

Name of family doctor _____   When last seen? _____

Do you smoke? _____   If yes, how many packs per day _____   Alcohol use? _____

Do you have   _____ Heart trouble   _____ High blood pressure

                              _____ Kidney problems   _____ Heart attack before/ after 40

Are you taking medication for cholesterol? _____   Blood pressure? _____   Other? _____

Do you exercise regularly?_____   When did you last eat? _____ hours

When you are finished with all your tests, please return to this room for final review of your results.

RELEASE:

I RELEASE _____ and the Health Technology Students from any liability as a result of my participation in this free Health Fair.

Signature _____   Date _____

Parent/Guardian _____   Witness _____

TEST	NORMAL LIMITS	RESULTS	FURTHER EVALUATION _____

URINALYSIS

Glucose	NEG	
Bilirubin	NEG	
Ketone	NEG	
Specific gravity	1.005–1.030	
Blood	NEG	
pH	6.0–8.0	
Protein	NEG/TRACE	
Urobilinogen	NORM	
Nitrite	NEG	
Leukocytes	NEG	

Clinitek: asterisk (*) indicates further evaluation

Urinalysis

Routine urinalysis is a basic test, but it provides the physician with a tremendous amount of information about a disease. This test can help confirm or rule out a suspected diagnosis. It is a routine test that is repeated annually or as frequently as necessary to evaluate the patient's health status.

HEMATOLOGY

Anemia

Hemoglobin: greater than 12 gm or g/dL   _____

Hematocrit: greater than 32%   _____

Anemia Check

The hemoglobin and hematocrit tests determine the oxygen-carrying ability of the blood. They are simple and efficient methods to detect any anemia. A patient is considered anemic if the hemoglobin value is below 12 mg/dL or the hematocrit is below 34%. Low values are caused by hemorrhage, pregnancy, recent menstruation, iron deficiency, or other causes that the physician needs to evaluate.

Erythrocyte Sedimentation Rate (ESR) = 0–20 mm/hr _____

Erythrocyte sedimentation rates are increased in infectious and inflammatory diseases, tissue destruction, and other conditions that increase the plasma fibrinogen level.

COAGULATION

INRatio   _____ INR

ProTime   _____ seconds

> Desirable 0.8–1.2 INR
>
> Therapeutic 1.5–4.0 INR
>
> PT = seconds

BLOOD CHEMISTRY

Glucose

        Fasting _____ (8 or more hours since eating)

        Random (hours since eating) _____ hr

        Normal 80–125 mg/dL (if 2 hr after eating) _____

Hemoglobin A_{1c}   **Desirable levels are below 7%**   **Result** _____

WARNING SIGNS OF DIABETES	
Type 1 Diabetes	**Type 2 Diabetes**
Constant urination	Drowsiness
Abnormal thirst	Itching
Unusual hunger	A family history of diabetes
Rapid loss of weight	Blurred vision
Irritability	Excessive weight
Obvious weakness or fatigue	Tingling, numbness in feet
Nausea and vomiting	Easy fatigue
	Skin infections and slow healing

LIPID PROFILE (CHOLESTECH TEST)

Lipid Profile	Desirable Numbers	Cholestech Results
Total cholesterol	Less than 200 mg/dL	
HDL cholesterol	Greater than 40 mg/dL	
LDL cholesterol	Less than 130 mg/dL	
Triglycerides	Less that 150 mg/dL	
TC/HDL ratio	4.5 or less	
Glucose	Fasting: 60-110 mg/dL	
	Nonfasting: less than 160 mg/dL	

Cholesterol

Cholesterol measurements are used to diagnose and monitor disorders involving excess cholesterol in the blood and fat metabolism disorders. These conditions often are associated with coronary heart disease. It is thought that lowering mean cholesterol levels can reduce coronary heart disease.

CHEMISTRY PROFILE I-STAT (Chem 8+)

Test	Test Symbol	Units	Reference Range	Result
Sodium	Na	mmol/L	138–146	
Potassium	K	mmol/L	3.5–4.9	
Chloride	Cl	mmol/L	98–109	
Total carbon dioxide	TCO_2	mmol/L	24–29	
Ionized calcium	iCa	mmol/L	1.12–1.32	
Glucose	Glu	mg/dL	70–105	
Urea nitrogen	BUN	mg/dL	8–26	
Creatinine	Crea	mg/dL	0.6–1.3	
Hematocrit	Hct	% PCV	38–51	
Hemoglobin*	Hb	g/dL	12–17	
Anion gap*	AnGap	mmol/L	10–20	

FECAL OCCULT BLOOD

Results: Positive _____ **Negative** _____

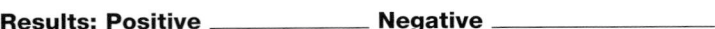

Appendix: Forms for Documenting Safety, Quality Assurance